ADRIEN ARPEL'S

Fast Beauty Tips

Also by Adrien Arpel in Piatkus Books

How to Look Ten Years Younger

ADRIEN ARPEL'S

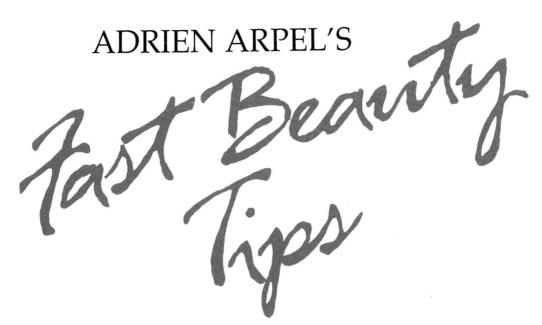

Fast Beauty Tips

701 shortcuts to looking good

with Ronnie Sue Ebenstein

PIATKUS

To Lauren

you are all things beautiful

First published in Great Britain
1986 by Judy Piatkus (Publishers) Limited
5 Windmill Street, London W1P 1HS

British Library Cataloguing in Publication Data

Arpel, Adrien
  Fast beauty tips.
  1. Beauty, Personal
  I. Title   II. Ebenstein, Ronnie Sue
  646.7′2′088042   RA778

ISBN 0–86188–393–4

Designed by Sue Ryall
Illustrated by Lynne Robinson

Typeset by Phoenix Photosetting Chatham
Printed and bound by Bath Press, Avon

Contents

Acknowledgments

I would like to thank Ronnie Sue Ebenstein, who is not only the best writing partner in the whole world but also the best friend; John Kubie, the chairman of Seligman & Latz, Inc., who never lets me down; Dr. Albert Shansky, without whose vast knowledge as to how a product is conceived and how it should be used this book could never have been written; Dr. Jeffrey L. Gurian, for his extraordinary artistry and skill in all things dental; Dr. Robert Auerbach, whom I can always rely on for the newest information on skin; Dr. Elliot Jacobs, whose expertise with collagen proved invaluable; Dr. Samuel Guillory, my ophthalmologist and one of New York's finest; Annette Green, executive director of the Fragrance Foundation, who knows everything about perfume and so generously shared her knowledge; and Joel Rubin, the chemist who helps make my professional products.

I would also like to thank my editor, Christine Schillig, for all her enthusiasm and support.

Introduction

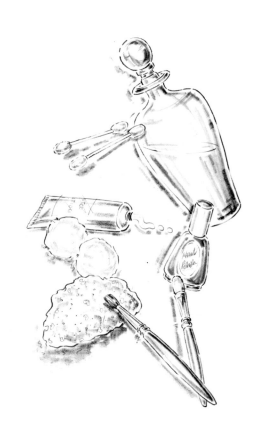

Dear Reader:

- *Upon finishing this book you will be exquisitely beautiful.*
- You will have thin thighs, a firm bottom, a flat stomach and stand-up breasts.
- You will have flawless skin complete with angular, chiselled cheekbones.
- The shine in your spectacularly healthy hair will be dazzling.
- You will be 4 inches taller and 2 sizes smaller.
- You will be envied and worshipped by all who are lucky enough to see you.
- As you ride into the sunset with your adoring prince (who will also come to you after buying this volume), you will thank Adrien Arpel forevermore.

If you don't believe the above fantasy, you and I have a lot to talk about. The cosmetics industry (and it's offspring, those I-Am-a-Great-Beauty beauty books) love to fantasize. But the ads and most beauty books omit one crucial bit of reality: Only a chromosome transplant will turn any of us into the 6-foot tall, poreless, cellulite-free, saucer-eyed, tiny-nosed creatures who grace cosmetics advertising. (I think the models are descended from an alien race. They certainly don't resemble anything found on my 5 foot 4 inch family tree!)

But cosmetic technology can help you look better and establish your own unique brand of beauty—if you know how to buy it, use it and *adapt it to your needs* so you don't waste a drop. Consider these real questions:

- How can you juice up that expensive night cream that's not working on your skin?
- What do you do with the moisturizer that turns the model's skin dewy and yours greasy?
- How do you enhance that supposedly ultra-zingy astringent that refuses to rev up your complexion?
- True, the lipstick is rich and creamy as promised, but how do you keep it from sliding all over your face?
- How to add new life to dried-up mascara? Lighten a too-dark foundation? Colour up your foundation to add some oomph to sallow skin?
- How do you really use all those sponges, brushes and applicators to give yourself a truly professional make-up?

I'll teach you how—with specific hints, tips and product transformations that will show you how to buy mistake-free cosmetics for the rest of your life, how to correct the mistakes already sitting on your make-up shelf, how to use everything you buy and make to give yourself an individual, self-styled beauty.

And I'll do it with a completely new kind of beauty book.

Your grandmother, mother and probably even you have bought household hints books that tell you what to do when ice cream or blood gets on little Georgie's school uniform.

But where do you look when problems relating to your personal appearance need a fast fix? Typical hint collections·tell you what to add to stretch a meatloaf, not how to stretch a night cream. You've read ad nauseam about six ways to whiten your porcelain sink, but not how to get rid of the plumber's hands that result from your do-it-yourself efforts. You've been taught how to get oils off your pillowcase, but not how to keep the costly oils in place on your skin at night.

That's why I think it's time for a new self-help beauty shortcut collection. I'm going to give you fast tips that will help you keep *yourself* sparkling.

I hope you'll use this book as you would any classic reference book. After a thorough read, refer back to it whenever you have a specific beauty problem that needs solving. There are tips for every age and stage of a woman's beauty life.

No, you won't be able to transform yourself into a flawless cover girl (even genetic engineers haven't reached that goal yet), but you will never make a beauty mistake again—no thrown-out products, no wrongly-applied make-up or treatments and no pages devoted to Cleopatra's beauty secrets or this year's TV sensation's reminiscences about her 18-inch waist.

How's that for beauty reality you can work with?

1
Preparation

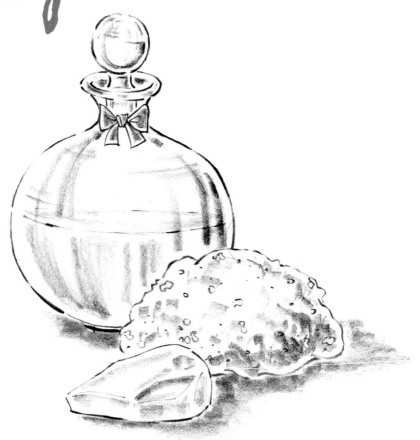

Most women really don't know what goes into the skin treatment products they buy, or how to use them properly. Treatment mistakes are made by even the most experienced of cosmetics consumers, yet these products are often the most expensive to buy and replace.

Today the cosmetics industry has the technology to make some very effective skin-workers, but women must learn to buy the right ones and use them properly. If you've bought some that aren't right for you, this chapter will tell you how to make them right—how to adapt and use the moisturizers, night creams, astringents, masks, wrinkle sticks, blackhead pastes, blemish serums, skin sloughers and more that you already have. Or, should you be inclined, there are several simple skin-worker formulas you can make for pennies.

Face creams to suit you

Is your face cream too thin, too rich, lacking in protein? Or maybe you just want to make it last longer, or learn how to use it correctly. Here's a fast tip for creamophiles and moisturizer fans.

MAKE A PROTEIN FACE CREAM

There's an excellent pure protein source right in your supermarket dairy counter. It's called whey, and you find it in cottage cheese. Strain the cottage cheese through a cheesecloth; that hazy-looking grey liquid that separates out is very rich whey protein. In the palm of your hand, blend 1 teaspoon of whey and enough cream to make a one-night dose.

NIGHT CREAMS THAT MAKE YOU SWEAT

Blame it on the greenhouse effect: A too-rich cream leaves a blanket or coating that holds heat within your body, so your apocrine (sweat) glands become very active. If you have this problem, avoid creams with a high wax content.

JUICING UP YOUR NIGHT CREAM

Are you ready to give up your night cream because you feel it no longer works? 'Additives' isn't a four-letter word when you

11

add 4 drops of liquid lecithin or aloe vera gel to 2 ounces of that lacklustre cream.

FACE CREAMS: SOME LIKE IT WARM

Does your night cream seem to lie on the top of your skin instead of penetrating? If you're losing most of it to your pillow, put one night's dose on a spoon and roll it gently a few inches over a low flame. Heat liquefies cream, making it penetrate faster and more thoroughly.

NIGHT CREAM SEALER

Canny Frenchwomen are known for their frugality as well as their attention to beauty details. Take a leaf from their book, and turn your best night cream into a European *penetrating* facial.

Melt, measure and mix in a double boiler 1 tablespoon of beeswax (available in chemists) and 2 tablespoons of lanolin. Let it stand until it thickens but is still soft enough to spread with a small paint or pastry brush. Then put on your night cream. Let it seep into your skin. Now brush the warm wax mixture over your face and throat, avoiding the eye area. The waxy sealer will harden, forming a heat-sealing shell helping your cream penetrate deeper into your skin. Let it sit for 10 minutes, then peel off.

VITAMINS FOR FACE CREAMS

To transform a skimpy night cream into an enriched vitamin skin treat, add ⅛ teaspoon of liquid vitamin C and the contents of a 100 mg vitamin E capsule to 4 ounces of ordinary night cream.

KEEP YOUR FACE CREAM GOING

You're almost at the bottom of the jar, but you don't want to waste a precious drop of the stuff? Stretch your supply by stirring in 1 teaspoon of mineral water or rosewater for every tablespoon of cream you have left.

AN EMBARRASSMENT OF (NIGHT CREAM) RICHES

You have a normal-to-dry skin, so you know you need a good night cream, but you'd like a lighter feel? No problem. Make your cream less greasy by adding ¼ teaspoon of glycerin per tablespoon of cream. Stir before using. Still can't stand the feel? Use that thick cream on your throat instead—or to soothe roughened elbows, knees or as part of a pedicure. Never throw it away!

OILY SKIN WRINKLE CREAM

Everyone says that if you have oily skin it won't wrinkle. Not true! It won't line as badly or as early, but oily skin will crease and droop eventually, so you do need a night cream—a *light* one. Salvage one meant for dry skin by adding ½ teaspoon of mineral water and ¼ teaspoon of baby powder to 2 ounces of cream. Stir very well.

DO-IT-YOURSELF EYE WRINKLE STICK

Do you dare to give him your 1000-watt smile while standing in the sun's glare? If the sunburst around your eyes outshines the noonday sun's dazzle, you've already tried sunglasses. So have I. Now try this:

> *1 tsp. beeswax (found in chemists)*
> *½ tsp. cocoa butter*
> *½ tsp. lanolin*
> *1½ tsp. petroleum jelly*
> *1 tbsp. + 2 tsp. safflower oil*
> *2 drops vitamin E oil*
> *2 tsp. white candle wax (from ordinary candles found in grocery shops)*

Melt all ingredients *before* measuring. Heat together in a double boiler until thoroughly mixed. With baby oil, *lightly* grease the inside of an empty, clean lipstick case with the base rolled down all the way. Pour the liquid into the case and let stand at room temperature for 1 hour. Refrigerate. Put any extra in a clean, empty lip gloss pot, let stand for one hour and refrigerate.

S-T-R-E-T-C-H YOUR MOISTURIZER

You're travelling, you can't get to the shops and your moisturizer is running low. What to do? For every ounce of product add 1 ounce of water. Although your moisturizer will appear thinner, it will work perfectly.

PLUMP UP YOUR MOISTURIZER

If the moisturizer you've bought doesn't seem creamy enough, don't toss it out—enhance it. For every tablespoon of moisturizer, stir in ¼ teaspoon of melted cocoa butter.

Tinglers

No, you can't splash on an after-shave to wake up your face. But you can go any man one better with astringents. They do more than rev up your skin—they make it look better, too.

HOW TO 'GENTLE' YOUR ASTRINGENT

If your astringent stings your skin when all you want is a nice zing, it's too strong. For every ounce in the bottle, add 1 tablespoon of rosewater or mineral water.

FRESHENER TOO WEAK TO TIGHTEN PORES?

If the descriptive word 'mild' on your freshener's label is an understatement, add just ½ teaspoon ethyl alcohol to each ounce of product and watch your face rev up.

SHRINKING LARGE PORES

You can't 'close' pores once and forever, but you can give skin the temporary illusion of poreless peerlessness (how about before a big evening out?) with the following hot-and-cold pore-shrinking bombardment.

Pour 3 ounces of inexpensive white wine and 3 ounces of witch hazel into a pot. Bring to a boil, remove pot from heat and steam your face for 5 minutes to dislodge impurities from pores.

To steam: Drape a large towel over both your head and the pot, making a tent. Don't put your face too close to the water. You want to steam, not scald!

When the brew has cooled, transfer it to a sterile atomizer or spray bottle and spray your face. Now add 1 teaspoon of liquid vitamin C (ascorbic acid, a good astringent) and refrigerate. When cold, remove from fridge, shake gently and apply to your face with cotton balls for a final temporary tightening. Keep the remaining mix refrigerated and use whenever needed.

Don't worry if your formula looks less than perfect. You're not a chemist and your output won't rival the store-bought variety in texture and appearance. But it will work.

SHINE STOPPER/OIL BLOTTER

If you have oily skin but you need (or want) to wear make-up all the time, boost your freshener as suggested above and carry 1 or 2 ounces with you in a plastic bottle, along with cotton balls. Blot freshener *gently* over oily areas when shine starts peeking through. Dot on a light sprinkling of face powder over newly 'blotted' make-up.

Skin annoyances and how to fix them

SHOW-NO-MERCY PIMPLE SERUM

Add a pinch of alum (found in chemists) and 2 ounces of witch hazel. Shake well. Apply to your face and allow to dry. Leave the serum on all day with or without make-up.

QUICK PIMPLE FIXERS

If you have no time to prepare your own serum, a Q-Tip dipped in witch hazel is a time-honoured alternative. To decimate a pimple overnight, dab on calamine lotion.

TAKE THE RED OUT OF A BLEMISH OR MARK

Combine 1 tablespoon of lemon juice with 1 tablespoon of salt. Apply the mixture directly to the reddened area, and leave it on 10 minutes. Rinse.

WORLD'S SIMPLEST SLOUGH TECHNIQUE

Everyone (except acne sufferers) should remove the dead cells that clog the skin's surface, giving it a dull cast. It's so easy when you mix ½ teaspoon of powdered Siberian ginseng (found in health food stores) into 1 tablespoon of your favourite cream. Apply to damp skin with small circular motions, then wipe off with cotton balls. Continue as part of your regular cleansing routine.

CLEANSING GRAIN SOAP FOR WHITEHEADS

If nose and chin whiteheads have become your face's constant companion, you need specialized soap therapy. Shave 2 ounces of quality soap (your potato peeler will work fastest) into a double boiler containing 2 ounces of water. Let soap shavings melt over low heat, stirring with water until a thickened consistency is reached. Remove from stove and add 1 ounce of soya granules (found in health food stores). Mix well. When mixture is cool enough to handle but still soft, coat your palms with any vegetable oil and work the mix into two balls of soap. Dampen the whitehead-covered area, rub the soap gently into it, then wash as usual. This soap works like cleansing grains to open and remove whiteheads.

30-SECOND NIGHT RITUAL FOR A BROKEN-OUT DAY SKIN

A few pimples are insufficient cause for abandoning your night cream. Just dab a Q-Tip dipped in calamine lotion on your blemishes, let dry, then cream the rest of your face as usual. The calamine will keep the cream from sliding onto pimples.

GODSEND FOR AN OILY NOSE

If you can tell the time of day by the amount of oil-breakthrough on your nose, yet the rest of your make-up is still matte perfection, you're a candidate for a nose mask. Mix together the following ingredients (all found in chemists):

½ tsp. fine-grind pumice
¼ tsp. alum
enough witch hazel to make a paste (about ¼ tsp.)

Spread the mixture on your nose. Leave it in place about 3 minutes for super blotting action. Rinse with cool water.

UPPER BODY BREAKOUTS

When you want to wear a low-cut dress to show off sexy shoulders and bustline, but your skin looks ravaged, a medicinal-type paste is just what the beauty doctor orders. To make your upper body paste, mix:

1 tbsp. epsom salts
1 tsp. bentonite
 (a mineral found in chemists)
1 tsp. ginseng powder
 (found in health food stores)
¼ tsp. alum
½ tbsp. rubbing alcohol (if necessary,
 add alcohol—¼ tsp. or at a time—
 until you get the paste consistency
 you prefer)

Spread paste on the affected area, cover with gauze and leave in place 10 minutes. Rub it off with wet gauze for slightly abrasive action. Rinse.

FOOL-THE-EYE BLEMISH CAMOUFLAGE

Is just one pimple marring the effect of your low-cut sleeveless gown? Colour it with brown or black eyebrow pencil for an instant beauty mark!

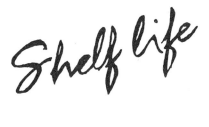

Which products last longest? What are the commonly used preservatives? How can you increase your product's shelf life? Here, a short look at cosmetic longevity.

PRESERVATIVES POLICY

1 Products without water last practically forever. Conversely, the higher the water content of a product the sooner it will spoil. Since bacteria find water, rather than other more exotic ingredients, to be the most fertile breeding ground, oil-based and glycerin make-ups have a longer 'fresh' life.
2 Glycerin is a preservative in itself (it's biocidal—a bacteria killer) and has a high longevity. Because it destroys bacteria, glycerin is generally good for problem skin.
3 Cosmetics with alcohol are long-lived because alcohol is a good germ killer. But it is drying to the skin.

4 Treatment products and cosmetics sold by major manufacturers (with or without water) contain preservatives so they won't need refrigeration. They should last up to two years (exception: eye make-up, see Chapter 5).
5 If you're an infrequent user, buy products in small sizes.
6 Do-it-yourself formulas should be refrigerated (cold inhibits germ growth and multiplication), made in small batches and used within a short time.

PRESERVATIVES NAME GAME

When you're trying to decipher cosmetic ingredient labels, it may help to know that the following scary-sounding words are all commonly used preservatives: methylparaben, propylparaben, butylparaben, potassium sorbate, quaternium-15, dehydroacetic acid. In fact, the paraben products heading the list are all derived from benzoic acid, a *natural* substance chemically treated to fight bacteria.

HOW YOU CAN INCREASE PRODUCT SHELF LIFE

1 Keep your fingers out! Any time you dip your fingers into a cream, lotion or powder you're reinoculating it with bacteria. Use sponges and applicators whenever possible and wash them frequently.
2 Store in a dark, dry place with lids screwed on tight.
3 Keep the paper, plastic disc or seal and always replace it after using. Air circulating inside the jar will help breed bacteria; the disc cuts down on air circulation.

IF YOU'RE ALLERGY-PRONE . . .

Buy cosmetics in tubes whenever possible. All products packaged in wide-mouth jars are more susceptible to invasion by bacteria.

WHEN YOU SUDDENLY DEVELOP A SENSITIVITY . . .

Immediately throw all your brushes, sponges and applicators into the wastebasket. Use throw-away Q-Tips and cotton balls, and introduce one new product back at a time until you identify the culprit. When your irritation clears up, you can buy new supplies.

Face cleansing

While children between the ages of toddlerhood and puberty are loath to perform basic cleansing rituals, somewhere during the teen years young girls finally realize the connection between cleanliness and good skin. And some of us haven't changed our cleansing routines since then. Here are a few facts and tips to bring you up to date.

COLD CREAM VS. CLEANSING CREAM

Cold cream has been around practically forever. It's said the Greek physician Galen (A.D. *c*.130–*c*.200)) whipped up the first beeswax-based make-up remover. And beeswax is still a main ingredient in cold cream, along with mineral oil, borax and water. Together they form a high-fat, high-alkali soap emulsion designed to dissolve everything from dirt to grease paint—and make-up. To counteract the greasiness and alkalinity, follow your cold cream rub with a water-soluble nongreasy cleansing cream application.

If you wear make-up, you need the old One-Two. *One:* the grease-cutting properties of cold cream to remove make-up. *Two:* the gentle action of a cleansing cream to remove all traces of the cold cream.

SOAP PROBLEMS

Soap is basically made from emollient oils and alkaline substances. A few of the most common emollients are lanolin, coconut, olive, peanut, soybean and palm oils—and they're *not* the problem. Rather, it's the alkaline cleansing agents such as sodium hydroxide or potassium hydroxide that can irritate skin. I prefer using a good cleansing cream.

SENSITIVE SKIN CLEANSER

Some of my most beautiful customers have thin, translucent skin that transcends puberty, divorce and problem children with nary a breakout. This flawless complexion is a gift from God (or genetically predisposed forebears), but it's often sensitive, demanding a soft approach to cleansing. I counsel using a light hand and that kitchen staple. Just warm it slightly to soften, apply generously with fingertips, remove with damp cotton balls or a soft (not rough-textured) washcloth.

Masks

How would you like 'new' skin in just 10 minutes a week? If this sounds like one of those too-good-to-be-true back-of-the-magazine ads (you know, the ones that promise you can lose 30 pounds while you sleep), you're right. But if you add the proper masks to your beauty routine and learn how to improve the masks you already have, I can promise you *noticeably* better skin.

THE THROAT MOISTURIZING MASK

People think I'm some sort of witch because I can accurately guess their ages without staring rudely at their faces. My less-than-magic trick: I zero in on a wrinkly, crepey throat—a definite giveaway. But you can trick me if you apply this moisturizing throat mask once or twice a week for 10 minutes:

1 tbsp. lanolin
1 tbsp. glycerin
1 tbsp. wheat germ oil (found in health food stores)
1 tsp. beeswax (found in chemists)
1 vitamin A & D capsule (25,000 IU vitamin A;
1000 IU vitamin D), pricked open, contents added
6 drops lavender oil (optional)

Melt and measure all ingredients. Place them in a double boiler, heat and stir until thoroughly mixed. When cool, pour into a jar and refrigerate. To apply, place a small amount on the fingertips of each hand. Sweep your fingers across your throat in upward motions from collarbone to jawline.

THE THROAT-TIGHTENING MASK: VARIATION ON A CREAM

If your throat is more saggy than wrinkled, melt 4 ounces of any night or cold cream and stir in ½ teaspoon of bentonite (a mineral, found in chemists). Refrigerate when cool. Apply as for moisturizing throat mask.

SOFTENING A TOO-HARD CLAY MASK

Since a clay or mud-type mask isn't a product you use daily, it may start to dry out before you're ready to toss it out. Make it good to the last drop by adding 1 teaspoon of mineral water to 4 ounces of too-hard/too-dry product. Stir together over a low flame to get it to mix properly.

INSTANT SKIN CLEANING MASK

Stroke milk of magnesia on your face with cotton balls (avoid eye area). Leave on 10 minutes. Remove with a warm washcloth and apply moisturizer.

REJUVENATING A TOO WATERY/TOO MUSHY MASK OR SCRUB

If your mask is no longer thick enough, you can add body by stirring in 1 teaspoon of baby powder per 4 ounces of product. You may have to do your stirring over a low flame to get both elements to mix properly.

INSTANT PORE REFINING CLAY MASK

Many expensive clay masks produced by major cosmetics houses have as their main ingredient bentonite, fuller's earth or kaolin. Buy any one of the trio (check chemists or health food stores), mix with water to form a spreadable paste and you're in business. These are strong masks suitable for oily skins. Leave them on for just 3 minutes to start, until you see how they affect your skin. Remove with a cool wet cloth.

Acne

ACNE AIDS

When buying over-the-counter acne preparations, understand what the ingredients do. Benzol peroxide is a drying, antibacterial agent. It comes in strengths ranging from 2.5 to 10 per cent. Dermatologists often prescribe it in 20 per cent concentration, and many of them now believe it is the only effective non-prescription agent.

Alcohol is another drying agent. Sulphur, salicylic acid and resorcinol are peeling agents you may find listed; they may offer some help if you have minor problems instead of acne.

If over-the-counter products don't work, or you have more than blackheads and an occasional blemish, get yourself to a dermatologist—there have been tremendous advances in prescription acne medications.

ACNE SCAR TREATMENTS

For anyone out there with scars from previous acne bouts, there are several methods for improving the skin's uneven surface. Options include dermabrasion (skin planing using a rapidly rotating wire brush); chemabrasion (skin peeling using chemicals); cortisone injections to shrink protruding scars; collagen and/or silicone injections. Your doctor should determine which method or combination of methods will work for you.

Exercise is good for your face too!

Give me your tired, your poorly circulating skin and I'll give you an easy-to-make face ointment, plus an exercise trio designed to get your face going. Why should your body have all the fun?

MAKE-IN-A-MINUTE FACE MASSAGE OINTMENT

You don't need to set aside an hour to perform a relaxing face massage. Here's a massage ointment you can use for a fast-face routine:

1 tbsp. petroleum jelly
1 tbsp. apricot oil (found in health food stores)
1 tbsp. olive oil
6 drops peppermint oil (also from health food stores)

Melt all ingredients together in a double boiler until just warm to the touch. Transfer mixture to a jar, let it sit a few minutes until it gels slightly. Stir and spread over your face. Reheat before reusing.

THREE FOR THE FACE

Not sure how to use your hands to relax and tone your face? Here's how: cover your hair with a terry towel turban or push it back with a headband. Apply a generous amount of your face massage ointment to the palms and fingers of both hands. Reapply as necessary, and perform the following massage exercises:

1 *Throat Toner.* Toss your head back and smile wide while opening and closing your jaws 10 times. Simultaneously, massage the right side of your throat with left palm and fingers; the left side of your throat with right palm and fingers.

2 *Cheek Shaper.* Whistle (or go through the motions) 10 times. Follow this with 10 sweeps of ointment-rich fingers in an arc from the corner of your lips, up and across cheekbones, out to earlobes.

3 *Forehead Flattener.* Cover your forehead from eyebrows to hairline with ointment-slathered palm and fingers. Push your forehead up toward your hairline 10 times without lifting your hand from your head. Now place three middle fingers in the spot between your eyebrows and massage in a circle 10 times.

Feel how relaxed you are!

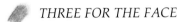

The effect of your health

No, skin abuse is not quite up there with alcohol and drug abuse, but good-looking skin is definitely a function of overall good health. Consider the following before you blame your face on heredity or the environment.

SKIN-DEADLY SUBSTANCES

If you submit your body to a steady diet of skin (as well as health) debilitators, you'll never have the glowing complexion you're working so hard to get. Resolve to eliminate (or cut down on) alcohol, coffee or other caffeine-laced drinks, cigarettes and fatty, oily foods. Overindulgence in these few culprits can lead to worn-out, sluggish-looking skin.

HOW TO COUNTERACT DEHYDRATED-LOOKING SKIN

To keep skin cells hydrated, and your face moist and young-looking, drink six 8-ounce glasses of mineral-rich water daily. You can use tap water if it's *hard* (high in mineral content). Call your local water department and ask for the number of grains of calcium and magnesium per gallon of H_2O (4–10 grains per gallon is hard; 11–19 grains is extra-hard).

If your water is soft (less than 4 grains) or just tasteless, stock up on delicious bottled mineral waters.

NERVOUS GIVEAWAYS AND THE B-BOOST

Does anger show up on your skin? If your neck gets all red and blotchy when you're in the middle of a confrontation, or you break out right after a stressful event, you may be short of the B-complex vitamins. The Bs—featuring B_2 (riboflavin), B_3 (niacin), B_6 (pyridoxine), PABA, inositol and others—combine to form nature's nonhabit-forming tranquillizer. They calm your nerves, helping to reduce the stress that can lead to tension breakouts.

Bs also help in the development of red blood cells and promote skin suppleness. But don't fiddle with the individual Bs—if you take too much of one component you may throw the rest of your B needs off. One B-complex tablet daily will end your dosage dilemma, and possibly lower your stress breakouts.

COLOUR ME RED: DILATED CAPILLARIES

Spicy foods do more than make me breathe fire—they also turn my face red. If you notice a link between blushing and eating, clear up those red-face blues by eliminating foods that cause facial capillaries to dilate (enlarge), giving you that little red spiderweb look: watch out for chili and hot curries.

ALCOHOL AND SKIN

My mother always said that people with lots of broken capillaries had a lust for liquor, not hot pepper. While that's quite an overstatement, understand that if you are a serious drinker, your liver isn't the only place the effects of alcohol show up. The skin, the largest organ of your body, also responds negatively. High alcohol intake may result in broken capillaries, and you may look dried up and withered, because alcohol overuse leads to dehydration—and it's water that keeps skin moist and supple.

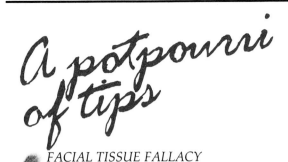

FACIAL TISSUE FALLACY

Which should you use for cream removal and face work—tissues or cotton balls? Save the tissues for blowing your nose. Seems the tiny wood fibres from which tissues are made can get imbedded in your skin, causing irritation (especially around the eye area). Cotton balls are best.

ON-THE-ROAD SKIN SCRUB

You can't cram your suitcase with all the beauty gear you use at home, but you needn't forsake sloughing. Filch a packet or two of sugar from the hotel coffee shop while you sip your brew. Back in your room, mix a small amount of the sugar with a dollop of cleansing cream in the palm of your hand and slough as usual.

PUFFY FACE WAKE-UP CALL

When I stay up past 11 P.M. my whole face looks puffy, kind of shapeless—like it's lost some elasticity. Here's a morning-after face-waker and toner:

5 tbsp. rosewater
1 tbsp. glycerin
1 tbsp. ethyl alcohol

Pour all ingredients in a bottle, shake, refrigerate. Apply chilled lotion liberally with cotton balls.

2
Making
Up

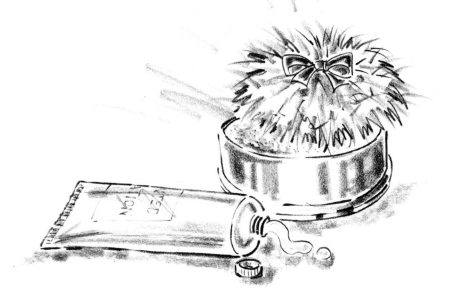

In a war zone, soldiers know the value of camouflage. Tanks, uniforms and faces are all masked; what's not meant to be seen is hidden from the enemy.

Well, I have news for you: Baby, it's war out there. There's an army of young girls after us and everything that belongs to us. Effective camouflage to hide under-eye circles, tiny lines, less than firm jawlines and puffy features should be part of your beauty arsenal. It's a matter of self-preservation.

You're barely old enough to vote? It's a good idea to learn early on what works for you and what doesn't, and how to camouflage those blemishes and facial flaws that beset even dewy-young skin.

You'll also want to learn to contour: It's the best way to give your face a sleek 'figure', complete with high cheekbones, shapelier nose, broader or narrower forehead.

Eye area camouflage

The dark circles under the eyes of an otherwise perfect beauty are probably the result of jet lag and too much Dom Perignon. Even though you and I are in bed by 11 A.M. and swill nothing stronger than carrot juice, dark circles, crinkles and bags can still surface. Here's how to make up for under-eye inequities.

 CONCEALER/CAMOUFLAGE/COVER-UP FORMULAS

Concealers come in stick and cream form. Sticks are available in a wide variety of flesh tones; creams in flesh, white and light blue.

Pale blue casts shadows away from the face (a trick first discovered by TV make-up artists). Naturally, when you wear light blue you must wear foundation over it—be sure to apply it sparingly in the under-eye region.

Don't pick white—your raccoon lineage will only be heightened. Do pick a product that will glide easily across the delicate under-eye area.

 ELIMINATING DARK CIRCLES UNDER EYES

Unless they're due to illness or diet, you can't get rid of dark

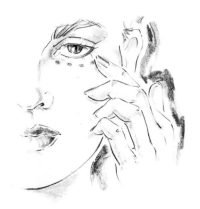

under-eye circles. They're hereditary. I've come to the conclusion that Darwin's theory is hogwash: My family must be descended from raccoons, not apes.

To lighten dark circles, use a concealer that is one-half to one shade lighter than your skin. Start your concealer just beneath the area where the dark circles begin, blending up and out onto the circles. Pat, don't rub.

CROW'S-FEET CAMOUFLAGER

To keep crow's-feet, whether incipient or full-blown, from looking like major crevices, keep your under-eye area moist at all times. Do this by applying a specially designed eye wrinkle stick (most companies make them) containing fast and slow-absorbing oils *over* your foundation in the crow's-feet region. You'll not only be keeping your eye area soft and moist-looking, you'll also be preventing more dry skin lines from showing quite so soon.

WHEN YOUR CONCEALER ISN'T WORKING

If your dark circles still show through, first apply light blue eye shadow in cream formula to your under-eye area. Follow with your cover-up.

WHEN TO APPLY WHAT

The order of things: moisturizer, tinted underbase (if necessary), camouflage cream/stick, foundation.

DARK CIRCLES AND GLASSES

Spectacles magnify your dark circles. Minimize them by wearing a lighter colour foundation down to where the frames rest, not a thicker cream or stick concealer; the lenses will only further thicken the appearance of your corrective make-up.

UNDER-EYE BAGS

Don't use cover cream or stick for under-eye bags; the lightness will just exaggerate them. We will discuss water-retention bags (the kind that improve as the day wears on) in Chapter 5. But if you have immovable fatty deposits under your eyes, tinted eyeglasses are your best camouflage. You can have lenses shaded lighter in the vision area, darker in the 'bag' (or lined) area. Pick a lens colour to complement your favourite eyeshadow, be it peach, mauve, grey—whatever. Many optical stores dye old lenses as well as new.

UNDER-THIRTY 'BAG' TREATMENT

If you are young and puffy-eyed, soak cotton in witch hazel, place it over your eyes and lie down for 10 minutes. If you are over thirty, this is too drying.

DARK PIGMENTED UPPER EYELIDS

If the natural colour of your lids has darkened with age, camouflage them with your skin-toned cover-up cream or a specially designed eyelid foundation. Most companies make the latter—they're natural in colour, creamy in texture and allow a less thick shadow application by eliminating the need for several layers to hide the dark pigmentation.

Concealing those imperfections

If you can't remove or eliminate bothersome skin imperfections, you can do the next best thing: hide them.

BLEMISHES

Even Hollywood royalty isn't immune to skin breakouts. When I make someone up for a movie, I conceal pimples by painting on camouflage one shade lighter than normal skin tone. Use a small brush, dab on concealer, then feather it out over the rest of your skin. Apply foundation as usual.

SCAR REVISION

A small scar or dimplelike imperfection (perhaps an old acne or chicken pox scar) can be hidden by building it up to skin level with your camouflage stick (make it two shades lighter than your foundation). Dot on five or six layers to thicken up the indentation. The thick application will fill up the hole a bit; the light colour will take away the shadow. Next, apply your foundation. This trick really works when small improvements are necessary.

CONCEALER STICK FOR FINE LINES

Vertical lines between brows, horizontal forehead grooves and other fine lines can be made less noticeable by lightening. Take an eyeliner brush reserved for this purpose, dip it in baby oil and paint over lines with oil. Next, stroke the brush across concealer stick, then across lines for precise placement. Blend it well.

What is contouring?

When you emphasize good points with light colours and minimize the less desirable with darker shades you're practising the art of contouring. The possible contouring corrections are endless: You can chisel out high cheekbones, narrow a broad nose, bring forward a receding chin. But to master this advanced make-up art you need a good eye, subtle application and *practice*.

CONTOURING COLOURS

All minimizing contour products should be flat 'taupe' brown, with no hint of pink or orange in them. Always use a taupe shade, nothing darker, or you'll run the risk of looking like you have a smudged face, on the other hand if you want to bring out your best features, highlight with light pinks, beige or white. And remember: Subtle contouring makes you look angular, a heavy hand makes you look unwashed.

BUDGET CONTOURING

You needn't buy a special contouring product. If you have taupe eye shadow or soft eyebrow pencil in the proper shade you're in business. A darker coloured foundation left over from last summer's tan can also work.

IF YOU'RE VERY FAIR

Don't use a special contouring product. You'll look more natural using a face powder just a few shades darker than your skin tone.

POWDER, CREAM OR LIQUID?

The general rule: if you have normal-to-oily skin, use powders or soft, chunky pencils. Skin on the dry side takes creams or liquids. Understand that creams blend easier than powders, but powders give a more chiselled look. So when it comes to contouring, you have to experiment to find what blends best as well as what feels best.

TO APPLY POWDERS

Use a long-handled (for better control) sable brush with a flat head. Art supply stores have paint brushes in all widths to choose from (or your favourite cosmetics house may offer a brush collection). Why a fat brush? Contouring demands long, sweeping moves: You need a brush large enough to hold the correct amount of powder.

TO CLEAN MAKE-UP BRUSHES

Mix 1 tablespoon of washing powder into an 8-ounce glass of warm water. Put brushes in and swirl them around. The debris will run off, and the powder works without abrasion. Rinse well in clear water and dry upright overnight.

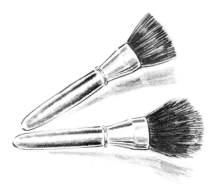

Fast contouring tips

Pick a flaw, any flaw . . . and I'll show you how to soften, narrow, shorten or elongate it. No, you won't make a less-than-perfect feature disappear (this is contouring, not conjuring!), but you will help it fit your face better.

SOFTEN A HOOKED NOSE

Keep a cheek colour well away from your nose. Stroke your contouring agent down the centre of your nose and blend well.

NARROW A BROAD NOSE

Draw taupe contouring agent in a line down either side of your nose. End it just above the nostrils and blend with foundation.

SHORTEN A TOO-LONG NOSE

Stroke your taupe powder or cream under the tip of the nose between your nostrils. Blend well.

BRING FORWARD A RECEDING CHIN

Highlight with pink blusher, white highlighting cream or foundation one shade lighter than the rest of your face. Blend well.

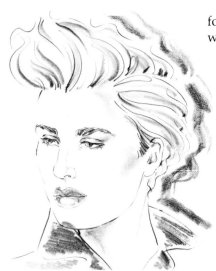

PLAY UP A SHORT NOSE

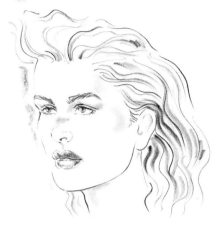

Cover the centre of your nose with highlighting agent, blending it outward.

DEFINE A SLACK JAWLINE

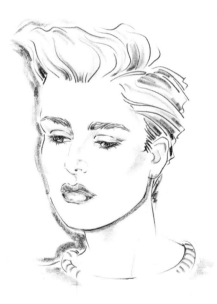

Raise your head and draw a taupe line from jaw to jaw. Blend well.

NARROW, SQUARE, OR JUTTING JAWS

Run dark shadow from below one ear all across the jawline and up under your other ear to play down square or jutting jaws.

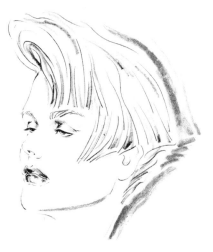

If your jaw is too narrow, stroke highlighter in the same areas.

ELONGATE A ROUND FACE

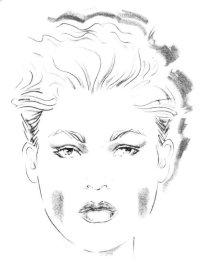

Draw two side-by-side vertical stripes from below your cheekbones out to the jawbone. Blend well. If you wear earrings, choose dull surfaces; shells, wood or dark-coloured plastics will make your face look narrower.

SHORTEN A LONG FACE

Add a bit of blush at your temples. Draw attention to your eyes with lots of mascara and the proper shadows. Shiny metal or stone earrings will also make your face look wider instead of longer.

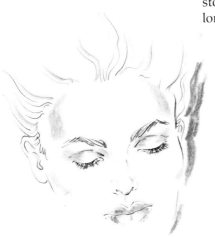

NARROW A BROAD FOREHEAD

Shade with dark contour to a width of two fingers from temple to eyebrow, down either side of forehead.

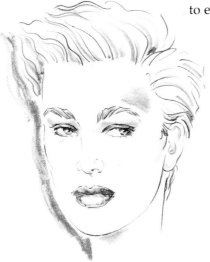

WHEN TO CONTOUR

The order of things thus far: tinted underbase, under-eye and blemish camouflage, foundation. The last is followed by contouring agents.

3 Foundation

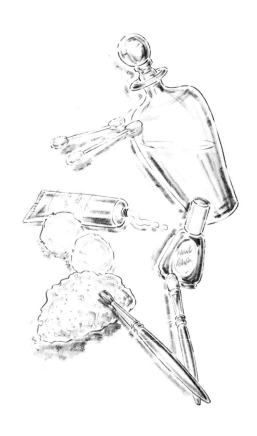

Did you ever have the experience of going out with another couple, taking one look at the other woman in your foursome and wanting to spend the evening in the nearest ladies' room?

But notice what happens as the evening progresses. After an hour her make-up begins to fade slightly and the goddess has become merely a terrific-looking woman. By the time coffee has been served, her foundation is streaking and you realize her skin has a few blemishes (not to mention enlarged pores). When they turn up the lights after the movie, you see her make-up has slipped away completely, and though she's not quite Dracula's daughter you wouldn't be surprised to catch her howling at the moon.

Her problem (and your ego salvation) afflicts many women: she picked the wrong foundation. As the evening wears on, it gets streaky, orangey, splotchy and starts to wear off altogether.

The right foundation properly applied can enhance skin colour, hide flaws. What follows are tips to thin a too-thick foundation; make yours medicated, darker or lighter, keep the shine out; apply it like a pro; correct your skin tone; avoid the heavy-handed look—and more. Remember, disappearing foundation is one magic trick you can do without.

Putting it on

FOUNDATION TYPES DEFINED

Gels provide all-over colour with a transparent look . . . good for giving a rosy glow or suntan effect.

Foundation creams work for clear, thin skin that just needs its colour evened out. They're very light, often whipped. Because they're thin, they are also good for lined, aging skin—they won't collect in wrinkles.

Compact creams are heavier, and they provide more coverage. They apply easily with fingertips or sponge, and are a good coverage alternative to liquids. Use them on dry, blemished skin, but not on oily skin (they have a high oil content).

Water-based liquids offer sheer coverage.

Liquid glycerin powders contain no oil or water, making them good for broken-out or oily skin. They go on wet, and are applied to a matte finish.

THE WATER-BASED VS. OIL-BASED TEST

How do you know which you're getting, since most foundations contain both water and oil? Take this simple test: put a little bit of your foundation on a plate. Add a drop of water. If it mixed freely, it's hydrophilic (water-loving). It doesn't mix well? It's a hydrophobic (water-hating) oil-based make-up.

MOST DIFFICULT TO APPLY

What is the toughest foundation to work with if you're not a make-up pro? 'Separating' oil-based liquids (the kind in which the pigment separates from the oil in the bottle). You *must* thoroughly shake the bottle each time before using, or an hour later you'll look like you need an oil rigger to remove the excess or as if you're wearing a full Kabuki make-up. If you need an oil-based foundation for your skin, use a cream instead. You'll get softness plus easy coverage.

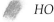

HOW TO APPLY

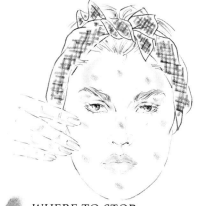

First, get your hair out of the way with a headband. Use the dot method: dot your chosen formula on forehead, cheeks, nose, eyelids and chin (a couple of dots in each area) and blend with sweeping strokes. Don't rub hard: you want merely to coat the skin—this isn't a deep-pore treatment. The entire face should be covered. If foundation looks streaky, reblend with a damp cosmetic sponge.

WHERE TO STOP

Do extend foundation from the hairline to down under the jawline. Don't foundation your neck, though. You'll just get residue all over your clothes. What if you end at your jawline but still get make-up on your clothes? Wait for foundation to dry, then blot with a damp, wrung-out cosmetic sponge.

COMBINATION SKIN

If you have an oily forehead, nose and chin, but the rest of your face is on the dry side, it's too difficult to use two different foundations. Instead, use an oil-free make-up over your whole face. Let it set. Then put moisturizer on a sponge and dab it on dry areas.

You've got problems

YOUR FOUNDATION IS TOO RUNNY

If your liquid make-up is too watery, you won't be able to thicken it satisfactorily. Watery foundation will streak and won't provide coverage because it just doesn't spread properly. Foundation should be at least the consistency of heavy cream. You might be able to use it if you're wearing a low-cut dress and want a bit of colour in your décolletage area, or to colour up bathing suit strap marks. But a too-watery liquid just won't work on your face.

TO THIN A LIQUID

If you want just a hint of coverage, and even your lightweight liquid offers too much colour, pour some in the palm of your hand and mix with an equal amount of salt-free mineral water. Forget club soda—it contains salt.

TO THIN A TOO-THICK CREAM FOUNDATION

If the cream foundation you bought is too thick, pour one 'dose' in the palm of your hand and mix with a little glycerin. If you're thinning the remains of a jar, use a coffee stirrer or swizzle stick (not your fingers).

ORANGE FOUNDATION

What's the problem if your foundation turns orangey-looking an hour after you apply it? It contains too much oil for your skin type. Correct this by adding talcum powder to help dry the product. If you add too much talc, use a drop or two of glycerin to get some of the moisture back.

Mix the talc into the foundation, but don't heat it because talc doesn't dissolve. It suspends in the formula and won't be lumpy or noticeable if you add small amounts.

WHY TALC? A VERY SHORT PSEUDO-CHEMISTRY LESSON

Talc is made from finely chopped marble, and it's the cosmetic manufacturers' best friend because it helps make skin feel smooth. If you look under a microscope, you will see that talc is composed of little plates that lie flat, coating your skin with a silky-feeling layer. Talc is also an excellent lightener.

FOUNDATION TOO GREASY?

Salvage greasy foundation by adding a drop of witch hazel if it's very greasy, toner if slightly greasy. Mix in the palm of your hand.

WHEN SHINE SHOWS THROUGH

Your foundation should see you through an eight-hour day without reapplication. If your face gets shiny and your foundation seems to disappear into your skin, cut down on your under make-up moisturizer (make sure you give the moisturizer a few minutes to seep into your skin before applying foundation) and wear a water-based liquid rather than a cream. You're already wearing a liquid? Switch to an oil-free (therefore very long-lasting) glycerin liquid powder foundation and eliminate the need for too-frequent touch-ups.

FOUNDATION THAT COLLECTS IN WRINKLES . . .

This is a problem for those with dry or no-longer-starlet-young skin. To cope, apply more treatment products to soften skin, and follow up with less foundation. You'll need a non-greasy collagen day cream, lightweight under-eye oil and, finally, moisturizer. Give each layer time to settle into the skin before applying the next product. Finish up with a very sheer lightweight foundation.

Colour ups

Few of us are born with perfect skin colouring. If your genetic cook programmed you to be too sallow or too ruddy, you can correct your colouring flaws with foundation.

CHANGE YOUR SKIN TONE

Many of us have either too sallow or too ruddy skin. Luckily it's easily correctable: prime your foundation with a colour-correcting underbase. I find that lavender works best to strip out many colour flaws. If you don't want to buy an underbase, and you have lavender eye shadow in cream form, blend a bit in with your moisturizer until you get a light lavender tone and apply it evenly over your face before adding foundation. If you have lavender *powder* eye shadow, scrape a bit off with a razor blade and blend the loose flakes with your moisturizer.

MORE ABOUT LAVENDER

1 If you have broken blood vessels or dilated capillaries, a lavender-tinted underbase will help mask them even if you wear sheer foundation.
2 Do you have hyper-pigmentation brown patches caused by the sun, the Pill or pregnancy? Add a little lavender eye shadow to your foundation and apply it to patchy areas. Let it dry. Apply foundation again over your entire face.

CORRECT YOUR SKIN COLOUR

If you stray too far from your natural skin colour, you'll wind up with a strange-looking masklike effect, so don't try to emulate fiery Latin beauties by applying bronze foundation to a Camille-pale face. It won't work. What will work:

○ to brighten a sallow yellow complexion—choose warm, slightly rosy foundation;
○ to tone down ruddy colours—choose beige or peach;
○ to colour up dark olives—choose bronze tones;
○ to enhance paler skin—choose ivory;
○ to warm up pale skin—choose pale peach colours.

Whatever correction you choose, make sure it's not more than a shade away from your natural skin colour.

COLOUR PATCH TEST

When you're trying on a foundation at the cosmetics counter, apply it on your face, not your wrist. These areas may have two distinctive tones, no matter what the saleslady says. Also, blend it down over your jaw—your under-chin area may be a touch lighter than your cheeks and the foundation has to work everywhere. Let it dry a minute. Can you see an obvious colour patch? If so, you've picked a shade too far from your natural skin colour. Try again.

WHAT BLENDS WITH WHAT

You won't know how versatile make-up can be until you learn to play around with it, recombining textures and colours to get exactly the products you need without investing in a walk-in make-up closet. Compatibility is the general rule: blend creams with creams, oils with oils, liquids with liquids, powders with powders. But, as with all rules, there is a major exception: You can blend powders into almost anything. Did you know that liquid make-up has *powder* colour compounds in it? Your imagination, colour sense and a bit of trial and error will lead you to the best combination.

IF YOUR FOUNDATION IS TOO BROWN . . .

Add some pink blusher to lighten it. Using a razor, scrape a bit of powder blush from the top of your compact. Blend it with liquid or cream foundation.

IF YOUR FOUNDATION IS TOO DULL . . .

Add apricot eye shadow for a peachy glow; pink blush or shadow for a rosy colour. If it's powder eye shadow, take a razor and scrape a bit from the compact; if cream shadow, add a drop. In either case, blend well with your finger.

FOR A LUMINOUS EVENING GLOW . . .

A drop of pearlized white eyebone shadow blended with foundation will give you a glowing shine. For more dramatic sparkle, silver, gold or bronze eye shadow can be blended in with your foundation *very sparingly*.

BUT FORGET LUMINOUS . . .

If you have oily skin, opt for a flat, matte finish. Pimples peek out from shiny surfaces.

SUMMERIZE YOUR WINTER FOUNDATION

If you bought a perfectly skin-matching foundation in March and find yourself with a June tan, become your own colourist. If it's a liquid, add a few drops of liquid bronze to colour the foundation up; for a cream, blend in some brown contour cream. If you really need a tanned look, check out the variety of foundations made specifically for black women. They come in a variety of shades to complement the depth and richness of black skin— buy the smallest size and add a few drops to your foundation.

WINTERIZE YOUR FOUNDATION

If you bought a foundation to go with your deeper summer skin colour, you can adapt it after your tan fades by adding small amounts of talc, a little at a time, to whiten and brighten the product.

Adaptations

You love your foundation, but it's your *skin* you hate? An occasional blemish doesn't mean you need a new product. With a few fast adaptations you can cover up a problem skin.

MAKE A MEDICATED BLEMISH COVER

Add 1 drop of liquid camphor to 3 drops of your liquid foundation. Mix in the palm of your hand and dab it on the blemish. To make sure you don't waste foundation, wash your hands, shake the bottle with your forefinger over the opening, and use the foundation that collects around the bottle opening and rim for your blemish cover.

MAKE A MEDICATED FOUNDATION

Skin broken out, but you still want to wear foundation? Add 2 drops of an antiseptic or your trusty witch hazel to your foundation dose. Mix in the palm of your hand before applying.

WHEN BREAKOUT IS A PROBLEM . . . A NO-WORK SOLUTION

Try glycerin liquid powder. It provides the ultimate nongreasy matte coverage that your skin needs.

Oops! Goof corrections

It would be nice to sleep until 11 A.M., then leisurely put on your make-up. But most of us don't have that luxury . . . we hop out of bed, take a quick shower and attempt to slap on foundation with our eyes still half-closed. The result: an occasional goof. But you needn't wash your face and start all over again. Suggestions:

CORRECTING UNEVEN APPLICATION

If your foundation tends to look streaky after you apply it, take a cosmetic sponge, dampen it slightly with water and stroke it downward over your entire face.

COUNTERACTING THE VERY 'HEAVY HAND'

If you're surprised when you look in the mirror (you're much more heavily made up than you intended), you must learn to apply less foundation. The best way to begin: Dilute foundation in your hand with an equal part of water if it's a liquid, glycerin if it's a cream. Then, even if you put on the same amount as usual it won't be as noticeable because the colour will be toned down.

FATAL FOUNDATION FLAWS

Bring your mirror to the window and scrutinize your face for the following errors:

1 Earlobes, eyelids and tip of nose forgotten;
2 Lips forgotten (essential if you're planning to wear lipstick);
3 Above-lip area not blended in;
4 Too much foundation collected by the sides of the nose and in dry-skin areas (i.e., crow's-feet);
5 Obvious demarcation line at jawline.

If any of the above exist, fill in neglected areas, wipe off excess and reblend with a damp sponge.

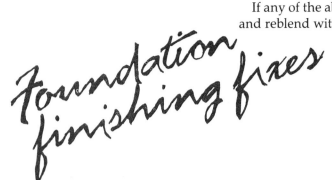

Foundation finishing fixes

SET YOUR FOUNDATION

When your make-up is totally finished, give it a few minutes to set and freshen your face with a mineral water-filled plant atomizer (the water should be cold—cold acts as a preservative).

Alternative: Chill your make-up sponge in the freezer and pat the dampened sponge over your face.

NOTE: 'Set' your face before doing your eye make-up.

'THINNING' A TOO-ROUND FACE

Once you're adept at foundation, you can use it to make *trompe l'oeil* face shape corrections. For example, a too-round face can be 'lengthened' by rimming the outer edge of the face (½ inch all around) with a foundation one shade darker than that used on the rest of the face. Blend the two together with damp fingertips or a cosmetic sponge so no demarcation line shows.

GOOD TO THE LAST DOT

If there's a little foundation left in the jar, add talc (or cornflour) and water to stretch it.

4
Powder and Cheek Paint

*'A little powder, a little paint . . .
makes a complexion what it ain't.'*

The teenager who penned that little ditty in my ninth-grade autograph book sure had my number. The truth is, I have yet to face a 'friendly' mirror without first creating the look of vitality that a little (or a lot) of blusher offers.

I'm one of those creatures who can jog for an hour, work up a respectable sweat—and still look as if rigor mortis has set in. Yet in just 30 seconds I can bring a glow to my cheeks that a month's worth of liver pills, brewer's yeast or raw egg shakes could never match.

I know that for many women putting blusher in the most flattering place is difficult. That's why this chapter will show—and tell—how to colour (and create) cheekbones, as well as how to stretch your blusher, blend cheek colour the models' way . . . and more.

Where to blush

WHICH CHEEK COLOUR FORMULA IS FOR YOU?

Let your skin type and foundation be your first guide. If you have oily skin and wear water-based or glycerine foundation, your skin will do best with powders, sheer liquids or gels. If you're dry-skinned, look for cream blushers or fat, creamy sticks. Combination skin is usually drier in the cheek area and can take any formula.

Let your blending skill be your second guide. If you're not good at blending powders, you may prefer liquids and creams no matter what type skin you have. If so, look for sheer foundation types and apply them in thin layers rather than globbing them on. If you have dry skin and prefer a matte look, you'll want a powder blush—just make sure your skin is well moisturized underneath.

THE ORDER OF THINGS

Cream, gel or liquid blush is applied after foundation, before face powder. Blush in a powder form is applied after face powder.

FACE BRUSHES

Here's what they should look like. Your blush brush should have a curved top; your translucent powder brush needs a flat top.

FOR BETTER BLENDING

If you see a line where your powder blush ends and the rest of your face begins, blend in with a slightly damp (practically dry) cosmetic sponge.

CREATE YOUR OWN POWDER CHEEK COLOUR

Take a touch of cornflour and blend it with crushed blusher powder for a lighter shade. For more dramatic shades, you can crumble deeper bronze and mauve powder eye shadow into your crushed blusher.

CREATE A PEARLIZED BLUSH

Mash a bit of highly pearlized lipstick and use it on your cheeks.

WHEN TO USE PEARLIZED BLUSHER

Save this trick for nighttime when sparkle is appropriate. If your skin is sensitive or broken out, skip the pearl. Though reactions are not common, it is a known allergen (see Eyes, page 64).

You can fake a gleam by applying a very thin coat of petroleum jelly to your cheekbones.

CHOOSING YOUR BEST CHEEK COLOURS

For a natural look, the fairer the skin the lighter your blusher should be. Pink and peach would highlight pale skin; reds work for anyone; mauves work better for darker skin. For nighttime, you can go a shade or two more intense. Bronze and earth tones work for a majority of skins except the most sallow.

NOTE: Never buy a cheek colour with a lot of yellow in it, no matter what your colouring!

FOR FLAWLESS POWDER CHEEK COLOUR PLACEMENT

Break into a big smile. Feel the fleshy 'apple' part of your cheeks (the spot Grandma would love to pinch). That's where you apply cheek colour, sweeping out to your ear. Blend as it grows fainter towards the earline.

FLAWLESS CREAM OR LIQUID BLUSH PLACEMENT

Break into a big grin. Place one dot of cream in the centre of your 'apple,' two more dots as illustrated. Blend them out to the hairline. To add lift to your face, add a fourth dot even with your eyebrow and blend it out to the top of your ear.

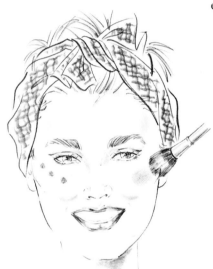

STOP BLUSHER FADE-OUT IN ONE STEP

If your radiant blush pales after an hour, apply a very thin coat of petroleum jelly first, and dust blusher over it. The jelly gives the blusher something to stick to.

CHEEK COLOUR AND FACE SHINE: LET THERE BE WHITE

To draw attention to cheekbones: after applying blusher, apply three dots of iridescent white browbone cream in an arc above your cheekbones. Blend it up and out for a subtle glow.

CHEEK COLOUR FACE CORRECTIONS

If reshaping your face with a separate contouring product seems difficult even after practice, and you'll settle for less pronounced corrections, you can contour with your blusher. You still apply it directly to the 'apple,' but you can adjust the blending angles as follows:

1 Add fullness to a narrow face by shading outward from 'apple' to earbone in a straight horizontal line;
2 Trim a full-cheeked face by starting on your 'apple' and drawing a diagonal line up to your browbone.

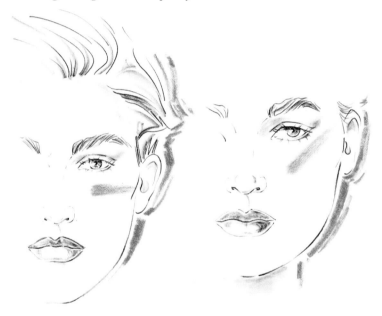

CHISEL OUT CHEEKBONES

You *can* create the illusion of angular, high cheekbones. Suck in your cheeks by making a fish face (luckily, make-up application is usually a solitary endeavour!). Feel the hollow beneath the cheekbones and place a dab of your contouring agent there. Blend outward, following the underline of your cheekbones. Next, apply blusher following the 'apple' method outlined above and blend with the darker contour line you've just created.

THE THREE (BLUSHER) COMMANDMENTS

You can improve your make-up look 50 percent if you remain wary of the following three sins:

1 Thou shalt not let blusher colour stray underneath the cheeks; that's for contouring only. Too much low-placed colour will give you a draggy look—colour is for highlighting.
2 Thou shalt not place blusher too close to the nose. Draw an imaginary vertical line from the pupil of your eye down to your 'apple'. Don't let colour stray past this boundary or you'll draw too much attention to your nose.
3 Thou shalt not apply blusher too close to the eyes. You'll only draw attention to any under-eye circles, bags and crow's-feet. Remember: Sweep the colour out (not up) toward your ears.

THE SUMMER BLUSH

Just as you can adapt your foundation to your sunrelated changing skin tones, you can adapt your blusher:

○ Mix your pink cream or liquid blusher with one dot of your brownish contour cream (or brown eye shadow) to get a more appropriately peached or bronzed suntan-enhancing shade.
○ If you already wear a peach blusher, just apply it in two layers to give a greater depth of colour. Or, forget your light blushers and stroke on bronzy eyeshadow instead.
○ If your pink blush is too light, yet your brown contour or eye colours are too dark, lighten the latter by blending them in your palm with one dot of white highlighting browbone cream until you get just the shade you need.

Perhaps powder

If you associate face powder with a Joan Crawford movie (I always picture Joan, Bette, Bacall, et al, pulling out a fabulous Art Deco compact for a quick touch-up), remember that audiences didn't call them glamour queens for nothing. Face powder (especially the moisturizing kind) is right for today, too. It puts a movie-star finish on your make-up like nothing else.

51

WHAT'S TRANSLUCENT POWDER?

Many women think 'translucent' means one colour that works for everyone. Not true! Translucent powders come in many tones, although most companies have just a few basics. If one company's translucent doesn't match your skin perfectly, shop around. You can also use baby powder if you apply it with a light hand.

WHO NEEDS FACE POWDER?

The oily-skinned woman is the obvious candidate, but anyone who wears a light, creamy foundation that slides off the face easily would benefit from face powder.

If you're dry-skinned and wear a light make-up, try a moisturizing powder. It won't cake and it will keep make-up in place on your face, even in humid weather.

POWDER TO CREATE A MATTE FINISH

When you want to create a polished, matte finish you can use loose or compact powder, but apply it with a puff or cotton square and press it onto your skin for greater coverage and more staying power.

LEARN TO 'SPOT' POWDER

You can actually use powder to help your contouring illusion. Consider this: matte, flat surfaces appears smaller; shiny surfaces appear larger. If you have a too-prominent nose and a narrow face, powder your nose to make it recede a bit and leave your cheeks shinier. I'd also leave a receding chin unpowdered.

TURN YOUR POWDER INTO A MEDICATED FOUNDATION

If your skin is broken out in spots and you find most foundations irritating, take a little bit of loose translucent powder in a skin-matching shade and put it in a small bottle mixed with your astringent. *Shake very well*. You'll have to play around till you get a colour and consistency that's right for you. Blend it well on your face. If you're working with pressed powder, scrape a bit off with a razor or with the handle of your brush.

WHEN YOUR FACE POWDER TURNS ORANGE

Make a thin mix of 2 parts cornflour and 1 part bicarbonate of soda. Put a thin veneer on your face under your powder. You won't see it, but the bicarb gives skin an acid pH to prevent it from turning orange.

PUFF WASHING

Your powder puffs must be washed frequently. Use liquid dish detergent or, for extra hygiene, use a cotton square or ball and throw it away after each use. When you use the same puff over and over, it becomes filled with oil and colour residue and can actually change the colour of powder on your face. A reused puff is also a bacteria collector.

POWDER TYPES

1 Baby powder is made from talc, a mined mineral that's actually a form of crushed marble. You can hardly see it on your skin.
2 Cornflour has no colour value. It's organic, made from corn and therefore is less apt to cause skin irritation than talc.
3 Most commercial loose and pressed powders are talc-based. Titanium or mica are added to make the talc opaque; colour is mixed in via iron oxides such as burnt sienna, burnt umber and ferric oxide.

5 Fast Facts for Eyes

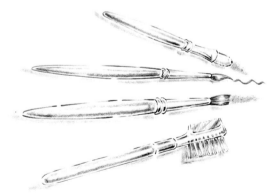

Without eyes for inspiration, most composers would be at a loss for subject matter.

Even in my sleep I can hum 'Smoke Gets In Your Eyes' . . . 'Spanish Eyes' . . . 'Don't It Make My Brown Eyes Blue?' . . . 'I Only Have Eyes for You' . . . 'Eye of the Tiger' . . . 'When Irish Eyes are Smiling' . . . 'Bette Davis Eyes'.

Yes, eyes communicate. But the reality of the message sent by your baby blues may not quite match the musical fantasy. For instance:

○ The fire in your eyes is really conjunctivitis, pollution, smoke or the result of one-too-many;
○ It looks like you have turquoise wrinkly-crinkly lids because your eye shadow has creased terribly;
○ He sees black spots in the corners of your eyes, where your eye pencil has migrated;
○ Your friends ask if you were mugged (but the saleswoman *swore* pink eye shadow trimmed with deep purple was right for you);
○ You look like you have just three fat lashes—your mascara is all clumped together.

Sound familiar? Then use this chapter to solve most of the problems those of us who pick up a mascara wand, lining pencil or sponge-tipped shadow applicator sometimes face.

Your eyebrows

FOOLPROOF 'EYE SPACING' TEST

Before you begin make-up corrections it helps to know if your eyes are too widely spaced (rare), or too close together. Take this so-simple test: Measure the length of one eye. Measure the space between your eyes (over the bridge of the nose). If the between-length is the same as the actual eye length, your eyes are perfectly spaced. If the length between is smaller, your eyes are too close together.

55

SKINNY EYEBROWS

You may love the skinny-browed, exotic, '30s movie star look of today, but will you still love it tomorrow? Narrow brows go in and out of fashion. If you tweeze your brows a lot for a long period of time they may not grow back, and your look will be dated. Remember, a crepey throat isn't the only age giveaway. Brow fashions change, and if you stick to an old-fashioned design you'll not only look out of date, but also older.

 BROW SHAPE

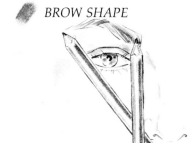

The classic two-pencil test is a quick way to determine how close to your nose to start your brow, and where to stop it. The arch should begin over your pupil. Place the pencils as shown in the illustration. If your brows end where the pencils begin, you're in good brow shape.

 AVOIDING COMMON BROW SHAPE BLUNDERS

When your brows are right, you don't even notice them. When they're wrong, the ensuing brows blunders can throw off the symmetry of your whole face.

1 Your brow should be almost the same width all the way across, not thick to the arch and skinny the rest of the way.
2 For a subtle arch, place the lift on a line even with the outer edge of your iris.
3 To shorten a long face, forget the arch altogether; a straight brow will 'cut' the length of the face.
4 To elongate a too-round face, make the arch slightly more pronounced.
5 If you have a short upper eyelid (you barely have room for one colour of shadow, let alone three!) tweeze an extra row (one hair at a time) from the bottom to open up your lid area a bit.

WHEN TO TWEEZE

After your bath or shower (the pores will be open from the heat) and before bedtime are best. No matter how careful you are, your skin will be somewhat reddened and irritated, so you wouldn't want to tweeze before going out, when you're in a hurry to put on make-up. Tweeze before you put on night cream, after taking a swipe at your brows with alcohol-dampened cotton to clean and disinfect them. Dip the tweezer in alcohol, too.

TAKE THE 'OUCH' OUT OF TWEEZING

- Slick an ice cube wrapped in a hankie across the brow area.
- Numb the brow area with a baby's teething pain preparation.
- Make brow hairs come out faster by softening them with shaving cream.
- Lay a hot washcloth over your brows for a few minutes.

BEFORE YOU TWEEZE

Once you've numbed your brows sufficiently, find your browbone. Close your eyes, stroke your fingers over your brow and locate the bony prominence. Open your eyes and keep rubbing so you see exactly where the ridge is located. Strays that fall below this bony ridge should be weeded out. Follow the natural shape and width of your brow.

HOW TO TWEEZE

With a brow brush or an old, stiff child's toothbrush, sweep brows straight upward to remove debris, then brush them back into place.

- Pluck one hair at a time in the direction of brow growth. Pull with a quick motion.
- First remove strays between the brows. If your eyes are close-set, pluck a few extra (don't overdo) to give a wider-eyed look.
- Next, weed out the underbrow area. Brush your brows straight up so you can see at what point the strays begin.
- Never tweeze along the top line of your brows.
- After you do a little tweezing, brush the brows back into shape so you can see how you're doing. Those midway checks help prevent overplucking.

TO SHARPEN DULL TWEEZERS

Just rub sandpaper back and forth across the tips.

THE DAILY BROW BRUSH

Brushing your brows is as important as brushing your teeth or hair. Once a day, brush them against their growth, then straighten them up with an old toothbrush to stimulate them and get rid of any old make-up or debris lodged there. Leave them standing straight up for a high fashion look, or brush them back into place. If you have a small upper lid or eye, the up-brushed brow will open up your eye area. If the straight-up brow is too avant-garde for you, try brushing the hairs near the bridge of your nose straight up, the rest of the eyebrow in the usual manner. It's a good eye-opening look.

OVERNIGHT BROW TRAINING

Before going to bed, apply a thick coat of petroleum jelly to brows. Then brush (using a brow brush or a clean old toothbrush) in the direction you *wish* they grew. After a few weeks, you should notice improved daytime brow management.

BROW COLOUR-UPS: POWDER VS. PENCIL

You may need both!

To fill in sparse brows, use specially formulated powder brow colour and an angled brow brush. Use short, feathery strokes, following the direction of the hair growth. Brush brows lightly back into place.

To draw on a better shape, use a well-sharpened brow pencil. Draw short, diagonal lines emulating natural brow hair. Then take your old toothbrush and brush through gently to soften the look.

Choose a colour close to your natural one. For lighter brows, bleaching should be done professionally. A too-dark brow will make you look as though you should be riding a broom.

QUICK BROW LIGHTENER

A little foundation rubbed into your brows and brushed through with an old toothbrush will lighten them.

Lashes

EYELASH CURLER: WHEN AND WHY

Look straight ahead into a mirror. Do your eyelashes grow straight down naturally? If so, skip the curler: you'd be going against Mother Nature and would risk breaking off lashes. For the rest of us, an eyelash curler makes lashes look longer, giving the eye a wide-open look. Curl *before* you apply mascara to clean lashes (you don't want the curler sticking to dried mascara; you'll pull out lashes when you remove it).

Here's *why* to use a curler: Lashes hanging over your eyeball create shadows over the eyes, making them look smaller. A curler gets the lashes out of the way, giving the eye a more open look. So not only do lashes look longer, eyes look larger.

TO THICKEN LASHES

Pat baby or face powder on your upper and lower lashes (topside and underside) before applying mascara to give lashes a thick, lush look. What about fibre mascara? It's not around very much anymore, and it's not for you if you have eye problems; the little fibres can drop off into your eyes. If you wear contact lenses, fibre mascara is a definite no-no.

TO MASCARA UPPER LASHES

When you apply mascara, don't hold the wand stationary. Roll it along your lashes, both topside and underside, from roots to tips. The rolling action helps deposit the mascara evenly onto the lashes and prevents clumping. Repeat two or three times, but let it dry between coats. You can use the point of the wand (after you've tipped off the excess) to prevent clumping. To do the topside, put your mirror on a table so your eyes are half closed and you're looking down. To do the underside, tilt your head back.

TO MASCARA LOWER LASHES

Hold the wand vertically and use the tip only to mascara one lash at a time. You're prone to under-eye smudges? Wind a piece of tissue tightly and hold it in place under your bottom lashes while applying mascara. Or, keep on hand a Q-Tip dipped in your eye make-up remover for fast touch-ups before the mascara has a chance to dry.

RESTORE DRIED-OUT MASCARA

Run hot water over the screwed-tight case. The heat may bring it back to life. Or add 1 drop of glycerin at a time. Mix with a skinny plastic coffee stirrer (the kind you get with take-away coffee).

Do not mix with your wand. You will ruin it.

WHAT COLOUR MASCARA?

Brown and black mascaras make your lashes look thick and heavy and create a becoming frame for your eyes. Purple, blue and green shades will not make lashes look as lush and are fake-looking. If you like the idea of coloured mascaras, apply first, then colour brown or black mascara on the tips. And, I'd save the technicolour tips for evening.

MASCARA TO BED?

Don't even dream of it. If you're one of those women who wears mascara to bed and then removes the residue under your eyes next morning with cold cream, you're causing more harm than if you went ten rounds with the reigning heavyweight champ. When left on overnight, mascara can become an irritant and cause the eye area to swell; or, bits of dirt clinging to mascara can get in your eyes. The result: a slight puffiness (or worse). If this overnight swelling happens often, the stretched skin will soon show lines. Besides, your cold cream is formulated to dissolve face make-up, not to remove mascara ingredients. So go for a special eye make-up remover, make sure it's fragrance-free and that you use it nightly.

EYE MAKE-UP REMOVERS

If you don't want to buy a made-for-the-eyes make-up remover:

○ Heat petroleum jelly to a runny consistency and apply it with your fingers.

- Put baby shampoo on a Q-Tip or damp cotton square.
- Try gentle apricot kernel oil on a damp cotton square.
- No matter what the remover, hold it in place over your closed eye for at least 30 seconds before rubbing gently, so remover has a chance to melt the make-up.

ANTI-WRINKLING EYE MAKE-UP REMOVER

Since you use eye make-up to enhance your eyes, it's a shame to botch the job by tugging to get it off (thus increasing the chance of premature wrinkling in the delicate eye area). Here, the easiest of non-tug steps:

- Gently massage a small amount of remover over lids and lashes.
- Don't touch the area until you've counted to 30—this delay is necessary to remove shadows and liners as well as mascara.
- Dampen a cotton ball and lay it over your eye. Whisk it off. Make-up should come with it.
- Alternative: skip the cotton ball and rinse with water.
- For stubborn mascara residue, finger a bit of remover directly onto the lashes, wait a few seconds and wipe them with a clean dampened cotton.
- Remove mascara that you wipe onto your skin with a dampened swab.

REMOVING WATERPROOF MASCARA

Because it's not readily water soluble, you must use a special oil-rich remover. Otherwise you'll have a tug at the thin-skinned area around your eyes. Cold cream contains only about 10 percent oil; you need a remover with at least 30 percent. Try pure safflower oil or a product specially formulated for waterproof mascara.

WATERPROOF MASCARA 'MINUS'

Some women feel that waterproof mascara causes their lashes to become especially dry and brittle. If you've noticed this problem, apply a thin coat of mineral oil to the tips of your lashes before going to bed.

Lining your eyes

Eyelining is one of the trickier techniques to master. But if you know how to adapt the tools to your own level of clumsiness you'll be surprised at how easily you can create a straight, fine line that rims your eyes without overwhelming them.

THE 'DRAG' TEST FOR EYE PENCILS

While lip-line pencils must be rather firm, any pencils you use in the delicate eye region should be soft enough to glide over your skin. If you have to tug and pull the pencil across the lid, you could create wrinkles. To test for drag, stroke the pencil across the soft pouchy skin between thumb and forefinger. If it glides without pulling, it should do so across your eyelid.

DRAG CORRECTIONS

Have you already bought one (or more) shadow or liner pencils that fail the drag test? Hold them near a match or lighter so they soften slightly (but don't melt), or run them under hot water for a few seconds. Apply as soon as they're cool enough. You'll have to do this before each use.

CREATING A 'THIN' EYE LINE

If you love liquid eyeliner but always seem to paint on a too-wide line, blame it on the brush, not your unsteady hands. Trim the brush a few hairs at a time with sharp manicure scissors until it's so narrow you can't possibly overdo. Or, go to an art supply store (taking your current liner brush with you) and look for a long-handled thinner brush.

LINER APPLICATION FOR THE UNSTEADY HAND

Have you always had a hard time getting eyeliner on straight and narrow? Don't use a liquid and don't draw a line! Instead, use a long (for control) handled kohl pencil in a dark colour and dot it on the upper lid as close to the lash root as possible. Now, play connect-the-dots: smudge the dots together with a Q-Tip.

THE BOTTOM LINE: FAST FIXES FOR YOUR LOWER LID

○ Using a long-handled soft pencil, draw a line outside and under your lower lashes flush with the bottom lid. This is easy to do and adds drama to any eye. Smudge the line with a Q-Tip to soften it. Line the outer two-thirds of the lid to create a wide-eyed look.

○ Rim your inner lower lid (the little platform right above your lashes) with blue pencil. It's a quick cosmetic fix for bloodshot eyes because the blue makes the whites appear whiter.

○ Rim your inner lower lid with a white for-eyes-only pencil to make small eyes appear larger.

'SHRINK' PROTRUDING EYES VIA EYELINER

Make too-prominent eyes appear smaller by applying a wide coat of eyeliner. The wider the line, the smaller your eye will look.

Eye shadow

THE UPPER EYELID DEFINED

For the purposes of applying make-up, your upper eyelid is divided into three parts: 1) the lid proper, extending from the lash base to the point where your eye socket indents (close your eyes and feel); 2) the lid crease, the indentation itself; 3) the browbone, the bony ridge above the crease (feel it) extending right up to your eyebrow. You'll be covering one or more of these lid areas with one or more shadow shades, depending on your eye shape and lid condition, as described later in this chapter.

THE ULTIMATE SHADOW ORGANIZER

Buy a palette from an artist's supply store. Take all of the shadows that you've received in those 'blockbuster' gift-with-purchase promotions, remove them from their cases and paste them (individually, according to colour) on the palette with glue. The products will be much easier to use and less bulky—and you can organize your colours easily.

FAST FIX TO MAKE POWDER SHADOW LAST LONGER ON LIDS

Powder shadows do last longer on your lids than any other kind. For super powder staying power, dip a sponge-topped or brush applicator in water first, then in powder shadow before applying. The colour will be a little more intense, a lot more lasting.

WHEN POWDERED SHADOW COLLECTS IN CREASES

To keep this from happening, dust over your eye shadow with translucent powder. If your powdered shadow is already creased, revive it by rubbing with a *tiny* drop of moisturizer. The shadow will look creamier, but that's better than creased.

Why does powder and *any* eye shadow formula crease eventually? We blink our eyes about every 3 seconds. This constant movement causes the problem. But unless you go into a catatonic trance, you can't stop blinking. You can prime your lids (see the next fast fix) to prevent the creasing caused by that other foe of permanence: shadow literally sliding off oily lids.

FASTEST SHADOW SET

Before you put on eye shadow, take a large blusher brush you reserved for this purpose, dip it in fragrance-free talc, close your eye and dust over your entire lid. The powder will give your eye shadow something to cling to; some will also 'land' in your lashes, serving as a good mascara base-cum-thickener.

IRIDESCENT EYE SHADOWS

Skip them if you have sensitive eyes (pearl can be an irritant for some people) or wrinkled eyelids (shine highlights, remember?) You need a matte look. For iridescent fakery, stroke a thin layer of petroleum jelly or lip gloss over powder shadow.

REMOISTEN DRIED-UP CREAM SHADOW

If your favourite cream shadow has dried out in the pot, add one drop at a time of water or mineral oil and stir. And remember, when you buy cream shadow, don't discard the little seal that fits in the lid; it helps prevent premature dry-out.

Colour choices

CHOOSING EYE SHADOW COLOURS

Never match your shadow to your eye colour. If you have green eyes, bright green shadow will overpower the iris. If you have blue eyes, bright blue will make your own baby blues disappear. If you want to stay in the same colour family, pick smoky, muted versions of your own eye. You want your eyes to stand out, not your lids.

Remember that dark colours minimize, light colours bring an area forward.

COLOUR SELECTIONS FOR THE NOVICE

You're insecure about shadow colours? Consider the following:

○ Taupe and grey are generally flattering to all eyes. Exception: if you're over forty-five, you need brighter colours.
○ Brown eyes: try plum, olive green, charcoal, any deep smoky colour.
○ Blue eyes: look for muted amethysts, violet, smoky turquoise (not bright blue), moss green.
○ Hazel eyes: olive greens, greys, apricots and bronzes, shades of gold.
○ Green eyes: use the suggestions for blue eyes along with shades having a hint of gold in them.

Once you become more confident in your colour choices and application, you can widen the spectrum. If in doubt, go for muted instead of bright tones. If you follow this guideline, you can use almost any colour you choose.

DARK UNDER-EYE CIRCLES VS. EYE SHADOW

Unless you camouflage dark circles completely, don't use brown or grey eye shadow on your upper lid or you'll have a hollowed-out eye socket look, suitable only if you're wearing widow's weeds.

BLUSHER AS SHADOW

If you're in a hurry, or prefer a healthy glow to define colour, a dab of blusher blended in your lid crease or on browbone works well, giving a nice unified look to your make-up. But don't wear it on your lid proper, right next to your eye—you might look like you have a terminal case of pinkeye.

FAST FIX FOR RED LIDS

Use light green shadow under any colour to mask out the ruddiness.

BROWBONE HIGHLIGHTER

A bit of shine in the browbone area opens up the eye beautifully. Candlelight or soft pink tints work better than white, and even those with oily lids can benefit from a creamy sheen here—the browbone isn't as oil-rich as the rest of the lid. I love pearlized shine in this area, but if you have sensitive eyes, of course you'll skip anything with pearl.

Master class on eye makeup

Now you need to learn how to solve those niggling eye problems most of us have.

TO MAKE PROTRUDING EYES RECEDE

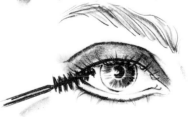

Since dark colours recede, you'll want to use a muted, smoky lid shadow—and an even smokier colour in the crease. A protruding browbone should be left bare or covered with your lid shadow. Don't use anything white or pearlized (matte conceals, shine accentuates). Surround the entire eye with eyeliner and apply three coats of mascara. Consider darkening your brows slightly. A dark frame will help puffy lids recede.

TO BRING OUT DEEP-SET EYES

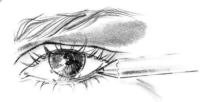

Apply pale or bright—not dark—lid colours near the lashes both above and under eyes. Apply smoky colour above the lid crease indentation (not in it) and blend up and out. Curl your lashes, apply lots of mascara, use blue eyeliner (which makes the whites of your eyes look whiter and therefore larger) to rim your inside lower lid only.

MAKE SMALL EYES APPEAR LARGER

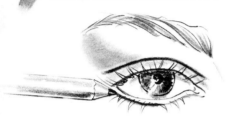

Start with a pale lid colour nearest your lashes up to the crease; a dark smoky colour in the crease. Repeat your pale lid colour or a soft-sheened pale browbone highlighter from the pupil diagonally out to the edge of your brow. Line your eyes with a smoky liner: rim your entire upper lid and half of the lower lid from just below the pupil out to the edge. Don't line the inside lower rim unless you use white, or your eyes will look smaller. Apply lots of mascara all around.

LIFT A DROOPING OUTER EYELID CORNER

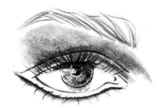

Lid, crease and highlight shadows should stop just before they reach the outer corner. Line under your lower lashes with dark kohl pencil, bringing the pencil upward at the outer corner. Kohl gives a smudged look without rubbing. Apply extra coats of mascara above the iris to draw attention to the centre of the eye rather than the outer corner.

TO ELONGATE TOO-ROUND EYES

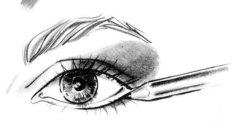

If your round eyes make you look constantly shocked, make them more almond-shaped by applying one shadow over the entire lid, starting above the inner iris and working diagonally up and out onto the browbone. Bring the colour around and under your lower lashes along the outer half of your eye. Line the entire upper lid and half of the lower lid with a dark, smoky colour. Don't use mascara on the lashes closest to your nose; do add extra coats on the lashes framing the outer half of the eye.

TO OPEN UP CLOSE-SET EYES

You've already tweezed a few extra hairs from between your brows, right? Next, apply browbone highlighter from lash base to

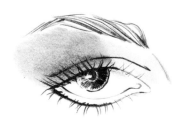

brow on the inner third of your lid from the tearducts upward. Then extend your primary lid shadow from base to browbone, covering the rest of your lid. Feather the primary shadow outward slightly behind the outer edge of the eye both above and below. Place eyeliner a third of the way from the inner corner of both upper and lower lids. Mascara more heavily the outer two-thirds of upper and lower lashes.

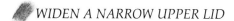 *WIDEN A NARROW UPPER LID*

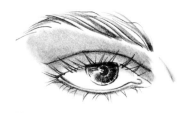

If there's not much space between your lash base and your eyebrow, use just one medium-tone shadow and extend it almost to the browbone. Use this same shadow to outline the outer third of the lower lid. Line the inner rim of the lower lid with blue pencil to draw the focus away from your narrow upper lid. Use mascara, but don't curl your lashes.

EYE MAKE-UP TO BED

Though it's not healthy to wear *any* make-up to bed, many women aren't comfortable with a new or younger bed partner . . . and no eye make-up. If you feel that the shock of your 'naked eyes' might be too much, consider cream concealer or shadow base all around the eyes; powder, nonpearlized eye shadow, applied not too close to the lid and tear ducts (perhaps just in the crease, blended out); or a touch of powder blush on the browbone. Curl your lashes and dab on a light coat of mineral oil instead of mascara.

NO-MORE-TEARS EYE CREAM PLACEMENT

Everyone needs a special lubricating cream nightly around the eyes to minimize lines and wrinkling. The thin-skinned eye area is susceptible to wind, air conditioning, sun (not to mention the propensity to squint and laugh). To insure that your eye cream doesn't migrate into your eyes while you sleep, first put the cream on the tip of your thumb and forefinger and rub the fingers together to warm it. This will liquefy the cream slightly so you can apply it in a *thin* layer—and it shouldn't stray as easily as when you glob it on.

Next, locate the under-eye socket bone with your fingers and pat eye cream on along this bony ridge. The cream will travel sufficiently to soften the eye area, but it shouldn't leak into the eye.

If your upper lids are wrinkled, dot eye cream very sparingly on the browbone just under the eyebrow.

PUFFY EYELID REDUCTION

The morning of my thirty-fifth birthday I woke up puffy-eyed, and began scheduling all my appointments after 11 A.M. By my fortieth birthday there were not enough hours left in the day to do business. So I got back to an 8:30 A.M. schedule by alternating these puff-reducing fixes:

○ Take a child's gel-filled teething ring, cut through the circle at a seam to turn it into a straight line, and place it in the freezer. When it's chilled, put it over your eyes and lie down for 10 minutes.
○ 'Freeze' a teaspoon. Close your eyes and cover them with a hankie. With the convex side against your face, press the frozen spoon gently over the eye area. This will help flatten puffs, and soften lines temporarily.
○ Use as little salt as possible in your diet. Salt causes water retention and will puff up your eyes.
○ Get up a half hour earlier than usual to give your eye puffs a head start on fluid drainage. When you leave the prone position, some of the fluid starts descending away from eye puffs, so you'll 'flatten out' sooner.
○ Sit up while you sleep if you must look bright-eyed at 6:00 A.M. A top model told me that the night before a magazine cover shoot she sleeps upright against *three* fat pillows so the puffs never have a chance to develop.

MASCARA REACTIONS

To prevent bacteria from developing and to avoid eye infections and allergies, replace mascara every three or four months. There is yeast, mould and other bacteria around your eyes. When you mascara your lashes, you pick up some of this bacteria on the wand, you then seal the wand back in the dark, cosy case and the germs multiply. Every time you reuse the wand, you repeat the bacteria deposit-and-return. Also, since there are no sweat glands on your eyelids—sweat kills certain bacteria—you're at a disadvantage.

This is not to imply that reactions are common. Far from it. But why take chances?

EYE MAKE-UP SHELF LIFE

One year is the maximum shelf life for other eye cosmetics. If your eyes are prone to redness or infection, replace cosmetics every three months.

 SHARING EYE MAKE-UP

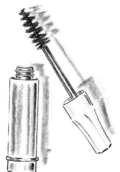

Don't! Eye make-up, especially mascara, picks up bacteria quickly. Avoid using a friend's, no matter what. Assume it is contaminated, and skip it.

OVERLOOKED ALLERGY FACTORS

○ The product that you loved at twenty-five may be causing a problem at thirty-five, not because your skin has developed a sudden sensitivity, but because skin gets dryer as you age—and dry skin gets irritated more easily.
○ Skip your brushes and sponges and try using fingertips for a few days if your eyes are red or itchy. Applicators should be changed at least twice a year—three times if you're sensitive. Maybe it's your brush, not the cosmetic itself, that is causing problems.

DO-IT-YOURSELF EYE ALLERGEN TEST

If your eyes are puffy and irritated and you're not sure why, try this skin test:

Choose a site either under your arm, along your inner arm or inner thigh or behind your ear. Wet the skin with cool water, then stroke on one of the eye products you use daily. Circle the area with a pencil and check it again in 24 hours. If redness develops, you're allergic. If there's no reaction after 24 hours, wash and repeat the process with another eye product.

Does all of your eye make-up pass the test? Keep your nail

polish off for a few days. Your nail enamel could be the culprit if you rub your eyes just after applying.

If you can't pinpoint what's causing your problem within a few days, see an ophthalmologist.

BEAT THE RED-EYE BLUES

Teary, red eyes are caused by the swelling of tiny blood vessels on the eye surface, which in turn can be caused by too much alcohol, eyestrain, lack of sleep, chlorinated water, allergies, etc. Over-the-counter eye drops contain vasoconstrictors that reduce the swelling in the blood vessels (decreasing redness) and antihistamines (to reduce itching). But if you use these drops frequently, your eyes may come to need them more frequently. You may find the time between red-eyed episodes growing shorter as your eyes become 'addicted' to the drops. It's better to find the problem behind chronically bloodshot eyes and cure that. You don't drink, smoke, go near the pool or have known allergies? Have your condition diagnosed by an eye doctor.

EYE MAKE-UP AND GLASSES

Take your prescription into account. If you're farsighted, your corrective lenses will make your eyes appear larger (and your eye make-up more prominent), so you'll want more muted colours. You're nearsighted? Your glasses will make your eyes look smaller. Opt for brighter, bolder shadows and lots of mascara so your eyes don't disappear.

EYEGLASSES AND EYEBROWS

Make sure your eyebrows don't show above your frames: you'll have a perpetually startled look. Your eyebrows should show underneath your lenses. And make sure the pupils of your eyes are roughly in the centre of the lenses or your whole face will look slightly askew.

CHOOSING EYEGLASS FRAME SHAPES

Pick a frame shape that complements your face for the most flattering results:

○ To shorten a long face, choose rounded oval frames or angled frames wider than they are long.

- To lengthen a round face, choose oval frames longer than they are wide.
- If you have droopy eyes, don't wear frames so large they hang down on your cheeks.
- Mask crow's-feet by choosing frames with temples (or handles) hooked to the bottom of the lens.

TINTED EYEGLASS LENSES FOR COLOUR THERAPY

Glasses can change how you see the world as well as how the world sees you:

- If you work under flourescents, make your office seem a little friendlier by wearing pink tints to cut down the harsh glare.
- If you wake up to a smog alert, wear yellow. It brightens up a dingy day, helps mask the look (if not the reality) of polluted air.
- Had a late night and can't bear that bright yellow morning sunshine? Blue gives off a cool, calming light.
- You love to ski but, oh, that reflected snow glare—mirrored sunglasses are best.

THE ONE SUNGLASS COLOUR TO OWN IF YOU'RE A BEACH BUNNY

The best all-around colour is dark grey, because it won't distort colours and is a good sun blocker.

TINTED CONTACT LENSES

It *is* safe to wear them if they come from a reputable optician. But understand that you can't turn dark brown eyes baby blue. Tinted contacts are best used to intensify the colour you were born with, i.e., to turn light green eyes into deep mossy orbs.

6
Lip Service

While you may never have the dream wasp-waisted figure, you can create luscious lips. But, alas, there are practical considerations: how to stop bleeding lipstick, use a lip pencil, curb lipstick breakage, soften budget lipsticks, cure dry lips forever, lighten a too-dark lipstick, create a custom gloss, etc.

If your lips could use a fast fix, you're in the right place.

Before you colour

The models in those cosmetic close-ups have gorgeous moist mouths ripe with colour that wouldn't dare stray over the lip line. That's because high-paid make-up artists never just whip out 'Plum Dandy' or 'Riot Red' without first prepping their lips. The keys: *prime* and *outline*. Here's how.

THE FIRST STEPS

If you want your lipstick to stay in place, and stay on as long as possible, you must prime your mouth first. Step One: choose a liquid, not cream, foundation. If you wear a cream base, it will run faster. Step Two: let the foundation set, then powder your lips so the colour will be applied to a matte surface. Even if you wear powder nowhere else on your face, wear it here.

LIP FOUNDATION ALTERNATIVE

If you wear a lightweight liquid foundation designed for oily skins, your foundation might not give you the 'cling' you need to get your lipstick to stay put. Instead, substitute a cover-up concealer stick. It slides on easily, yet makes a good lip colour base.

STOP BLEEDING LIPSTICK

There's nothing more unattractive than having your lipstick 'bleeding' into those tiny paper-cut lines around your mouth (or, if you're too young to have them, smeary-looking lips are equally unattractive). To avoid this problem, after you apply foundation and powder, outline your entire lips with lip pencil.

PENCIL POINTERS

○ Never buy a lip pencil without buying a pencil sharpener. A sharp point is indispensable for making a well-defined lip line.

74

○ Put your lip pencil in the freezer for 15 minutes before sharpening so the point won't break.

○ If possible, sharpen the pencil before each use.

○ In hot weather, store your pencils in the refrigerator so they won't soften: a firm point is essential for outlining.

BRUSH VS. PENCIL

When it comes to outlining, a pencil is easier to work with than a lip brush and it gives a more defined line. I'll mention a few other uses for a lip brush as the chapter proceeds, but it's not an essential tool.

V FOR VICTORY—AND NO-FAULT LIP-LINING

If you have trouble drawing a straight outline, put your middle and forefinger on either side of your mouth (fingers forming a V shape) and gently stretch. At the same time, stretch your lips over your teeth. Artists know it's easier to draw on a firmly pulled rather than wavy canvas.

THE LIP MAP

Here's the route to follow when outlining:

1 Start in the centre of the top lip, draw a line out to one corner in a nonstop, fluid motion.
2 Start in the centre and proceed in the same way to the other corner.
3 For the bottom lip, start in either corner and proceed with one nonstop line to the other corner.

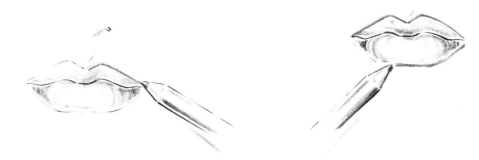

CORNER TREATMENT

If you're serious about perfect lipstick application, don't neglect the corners. The best way to fill them in is to stretch your mouth into an 'O' shape, brush your lipstick brush over your lip colour and paint over the corners using the narrow edge of the brush. Or, resharpen your pencil and use it to fill in the corners while holding your mouth in the 'O' shape.

TO BLOT OR NOT?

Never! You'll undo all the work you did. If you feel the need to blot, you've applied too much stick or gloss.

LIP COLOUR AND MOUTH SIZE

To make your mouth look large, wear light bright colours. To make your mouth appear smaller, wear dark or muted colours.

CREATING FULLER LIPS

If your lips are thin, build them up by applying lip-line pencil a few shades darker than your lipstick directly above the natural lip line. Blend so there is no demarcation line.

NARROWING FULL LIPS

Use a lip-line pencil a few shades darker than your lipstick. Apply it just inside the lip line, making the mouth smaller. Blend so there is no demarcation line.

CHEERING A DROOPY MOUTH

Lipstick can give you a happier face: Outline your droopy lower lip slightly upward in the corners and use a colour a half shade darker on your lower lips to draw attention to the upper lip. Finish by dotting gloss in the centre of your upper lip only.

TEETH WHITENING TRICK

If your teeth are slightly yellow, pink or red lipsticks (even plum or mauve) will make them look much whiter in comparison. Avoid browns and corals—they emphasize yellow tones.

Help your "yucky lips"

Peeling, dry, cracked lips are a disaster. But like most disasters of the less-than-comic variety, they can be prevented and/or cured.

LIPSTICK AS DRY LIP THERAPY

Did you know your lips contain *no* oil glands? That's why they're subject to chapping and parching even when the weather is mild. Lipstick contains emollients that counteract this natural dryness, so even when you're at home you don't want to go around with bare, unprotected lips. If you don't like lipstick, at least wear a light coat of gloss or petroleum jelly on your mouth.

DRY LIPS TREATMENT

Take ½ teaspoon of your favourite lip gloss, melt it and mix in ¼ teaspoon of either lanolin, petroleum jelly or cocoa butter, whichever appeals to you most. Store in a clean glass pot.

LIP MASSAGE

Chronic dry lips (you've neglected to wear lipstick or gloss on a daily basis?) need extra help. Take a rich emollient (lanolin, or petroleum jelly) and glob it on your lips. Leave it on 10 minutes. Wind a hot, wet washcloth around your index finger and gently massage lips in circular motions to get rid of flaky skin, leaving lips softer.

SOFTENING LIP-LINE WRINKLES

Here's a tip models use to keep their lip lines smooth: Add 1½ teaspoons of fine grind pumice to ½ tablespoon of your favourite cleansing cream. Mix well to make a fine powder. Work the mixture all *around* your mouth (not on lips themselves). Wipe it off with cotton balls, then apply emollient cream or your eye stick to the area.

SPORTS BALM

If skiing, ice skating and other cold weather activities are part of your exercise regimen, your lips need extra protection. Mix equal parts of lanolin and beeswax, melt in a double boiler, pour into small jar and stir. Apply to lips when cool. Reapply frequently as long as you stay outdoors.

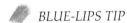

The whole point of wearing lipstick is to give your mouth presence, a feat that can't be accomplished in the absence of colour and shine.

CHOOSE A FLATTERING LIP COLOUR

○ Never try to match your lip colour to your outfit.
○ Lip colour should relate to cheek colour. A faint pink blush on the cheeks looks odd paired with siren-red lipstick.
○ Consider your overall make-up picture. If you're fond of lots of eye make-up, you should wear a noticeable (I don't necessarily mean flashy) lip colour. Example: do mauve eye shadow, kohl eyeliner rimming upper and lower lids, and three coats of mascara characterize your look? Then if all you wear on your mouth is transparent gloss (or nothing) you'll look like you forgot to finish your make-up!

BLUE-LIPS TIP

If your lipstick turns blue as you wear it, applying foundation plus powder to your lips first (to make a barrier against your body chemistry) might be a solution. To finish, rub just a *drop* of lanolin between your fingers and apply it over your lipstick with a lip brush to create a barrier against the environment.

LIGHTENING LIPSTICK

Last season's shade is too dark? Use gold lipstick stabilizer or lip gloss underneath for a lighter look.

MAKE A LIGHTER LIPSTICK

The lipstick that seemed right by the soft light of the cosmetics counter looks too dark in the harsh lights of reality. What to do? Take 1 teaspoon-sized chunk of lipstick, mix with ½ teaspoon beeswax and ½ teaspoon petroleum jelly and melt all in the top half of a double boiler. Put mixture in clean glass pot or small container. The consistency will be different, but you should have a colour you can live with.

LIP GLOSS SUBSTITUTE

If you don't like the sticky feel of gloss, but you do like the colour plus shine, apply powder blusher in a lip-flattering shade to your lips. Coat with a *thin* layer of petroleum jelly or honey that you've softened between your thumb and forefinger.

CREATE A CUSTOM GLOSS

Shave a pink, coral, brown or red powdered blusher with a razor and mix with clear lip gloss a little at a time to create your own custom lip 'stains'.

Or, cut the top off a favourite old lipstick with a razor blade, crush the colour, and melt it with petroleum jelly.

WHERE TO GLOSS

Have you applied your lipstick, and now you're ready to reach for the gloss pot? Use it sparingly. The totally glossed mouth is too difficult to keep for more than 5 minutes. Dot the gloss on in the centre of your mouth, both upper and lower lips, for a subtle shine.

THE NO-GLOSS SOLUTION TO TWO DULL LIP PROBLEMS

Problem No. 1: Even one coat of lipstick makes you feel that you're wearing too much lip colour.

Problem No. 2: You're over thirty-five and you notice that gloss travels faster than lipstick, and tends to escape across even properly lined lips and seep into the little feathery lines above.

Solution: Wear a lipstick with a little pearl in it. You'll get a low-watt shine without adding a gloss layer.

BLAME IT ON PEARL

If you favour pearlized products, understand that they break more easily. Pearly substances (mica, iron oxides, titanium diox-

79

ide and other inorganic materials) are very brittle. So if you're heavy-handed with any pearlized lipstick, cheek or eye colours, you risk breakage. Pearl is also an expensive purchase for the manufacturer (which is why these products cost you more).

Repairs

By now you've probably guessed I'm not in favour of throwing anything away, even lipstick. Here's how to make yours last.

HOW TO SALVAGE A WELL-LOVED LIPSTICK

Only a little left, but you hate to throw it out? Pry it out of the case with an orange stick, put the remains in a small pot over low heat, adding just enough petroleum jelly to give a creamy consistency. Melt together, stir and you'll have a pretty lip stain based on your favourite shade. If you have some old cream blusher in the same colour family, add it in too.

CURB LIPSTICK BREAKAGE

If your lipstick is always breaking, reshape it the way expensive cosmetics manufacturers do—into a wedge. Cut off the top with a razor blade. Save the tops—you can always melt them together for a new look and use as cheek colour, browbone colour or lip gloss.

Special effects and effective special fixes

If you're willing to go one step beyond, here's a quick collection of lip fixes you'll want to know about.

HOW TO PLAY UP YOUR MOST VISIBLE EROGENOUS ZONE

When I do a model's make-up for a photography 'shoot,' she's not ready to face the cameras until I create a sexy pout. Here's how: outline lips in a darker colour and use that same colour on your entire upper lip and the outer two-thirds of your lower lip. Fill in the centre of the lower lip with a lighter shade in the same family, creating a 'spotlight'. Blend the two colours well. Highlight the spot with a touch of gloss.

For evening, use the same colour lipstick on upper and lower lips and highlight the centre of the lower lip with a gold powder (look for gold-flecked eye shadow or finishing powder).

24-HOUR LIPSTICK

Forget it! There's no such thing. Assuming you're going to eat, drink and be merry, or at least mobile, no lipstick will stay put without touch-ups. If you want a long-lasting formula, look for the least creamy lipstick.

Or try a pearl lipstick. Pearls stay on longer because the pearl counteracts the cream.

UPGRADING BUDGET LIPSTICKS

Less expensive lipsticks often contain fewer emollients, so they may feel dry on your lips. A touch of clear gloss dotted directly on the tip of the lipstick before you apply it to your lips will give you a moister, better look for your money.

WHEN, WHERE AND HOW TO TOUCH-UP

1 The only acceptable touch-up you can do in public is on your lips. Excuse yourself if your face needs more work.
2 A quick touch-up involves slicking on a bit more lipstick. A total mouth re-do means removing the old lipstick completely, a 'private' job (but necessary if you want to avoid that thick, smeary look).
3 When old lipstick is off, you must once again apply foundation, powder and outline in pencil if you want a like-new mouth.

7

Dental Details

Unless you're a ventriloquist who has mastered the art of speaking without opening your mouth (sorry, clenching your teeth isn't good enough), knowing how to make up your lips won't suffice.

Your teeth reveal quite a bit about you, and what they say may not always be flattering. Yellow teeth with plaque build-up may indicate you're sloppy in your personal habits; visible silver fillings mean both you and your dentist don't know the most modern techniques; gaps between your teeth indicate Mother didn't take care of you (blame others whenever possible!); braces reveal you've come a long way, baby (see, I'm not completely negative).

If you still equate dental doings with an unending session with Torquemada, cheer up: The pain and drain (on the finances as well as the brain) are not as awful as they once were. Following are teeth (and breath) fast fixes you can perform yourself—and, more important, all the newest dentistry doings.

P.S.: You cringe whenever a photographer tells you to say 'Cheese?' Be sure to check out the fifteen photo fixes at the end of this chapter.

Seven tips for bad breath

Unless you're ill, you needn't walk around with a less than fresh-smelling mouth. The proof follows:

1 Eat regular meals. When you skip meals, bacteria build up on the tongue, causing odour. That's why BB can be an unwelcome side effect of dieting.
2 Brush your tongue and the roof of your mouth along with your teeth.
3 You really must brush your teeth after every meal. Leaving food in your mouth between meals is like leaving it on the kitchen counter for hours at a time—it rots, causing bad breath. (Keep a toothbrush and toothpaste in your desk at work.)
4 Careful flossing with unwaxed dental floss also helps. If you can't floss, try toothpicks, small sticks you work around and between your teeth to clean out debris.
5 If you want to indulge in raw onion, eat a sprig of parsley for dessert.

83

6 Follow dinner with a light mint tea instead of coffee for a nicer mouth scent.

7 Instead of store-bought mouthwash, make a strong brew of peppermint tea. Let it cool and refrigerate it. It tastes good, and peppermint is a natural breath sweetener.

Do-it-yourself dentistry

No, you can't use your trusty electric drill on your teeth. But neither should you leave total control of your mouth's dentistry in the hands of your dentist. Pick up the accessories and info you need to shout 'Look Ma, no cavities . . . gum disease . . . toothaches . . .'

GUM THERAPY

Adults can lose healthy teeth due to sick gums. The threat of gum disease, not cavities, is the reason you should see your dentist twice a year. If your gums bleed often when you brush, see your dentist *tomorrow*.

GUM MASSAGE

Wet your index finger and massage your gums in a circular motion to promote circulation and gum health.

TOOTHBRUSH TIPS

Did you know that one toothbrush isn't enough? Use one of the new bent-handled brushes for your back teeth and behind your lower front teeth, and a regular toothbrush for the rest of your teeth.

The bristles should be soft nylon. Hard bristles are now considered a dental no-no; they can damage the teeth. Soften too-hard bristles by holding them under hot water; firm them up *a bit* by running under cold water.

Dental gadgetry

Your chemist contains many inexpensive gadgets designed to promote tooth and gum health between checkups. Consider:

○ A dental mirror to see if your back teeth are really clean.
○ An Orapik to remove food and plaque (like performing at-home scaling).
○ Soft plastic toothpicks to get between teeth.
○ Various accessories that fit on a toothbrush-like handle (tufts, spirals, etc.) to strengthen gums, remove plaque, clean between spaces.

A potpourri of tips

TOOTHACHE RELIEVERS

○ If you prefer death to the agony of a toothache, especially the seemingly trivial (until it happens to you) problem of having a filling fall out, dip a piece of cotton into oil of cloves and lodge it against your tooth until you can see a dentist.
○ Hot salt water is good for canker sores, and so is Vitamin E oil (you can also rub the latter on lip sores).
○ Don't put aspirin near a bad tooth. It's an acid and will burn the lining of your cheek and gum.

STOP THE BLEEDING

You've had a wisdom tooth extracted, you're bleeding and there's no gauze in the house? Wet a teabag under cold water and bite on it for 30–40 minutes. The tannic acid in the tea is a vasoconstrictor, narrowing the blood vessels. (You might also try this fast tip if you've nicked yourself when shaving.)

HEALTH NUTS BEWARE

Don't overdo the citrus fruits, and especially forego biting on lemons. Too much citric acid can eat away at tooth enamel. Don't brush your teeth overzealously. If you brush too hard, you can get grooves at the gum-line and damage the surface of your teeth.

SMOKER'S TOOTHPASTE

Toothpastes designed to remove nicotine stains are abrasive; use them only once or twice a week.

TOOTHPASTE SUBSTITUTE

When you're out of toothpaste, brush with plain baking soda. It's a good whitener.

Say "cheese"

Because I must have my picture taken quite often, I make it a practice to badger the photographers for tips that will help me look my best. Top New York City fashion photographer Gideon Lewin offers these fifteen fast fixes for all of us amateur models:

1 Give your make-up a matte finish. If you're shiny to start with, you'll look greasy under the strobe and flashlights. If you're having your picture taken outdoors, a little sheen is OK.
2 In daylight, avoid direct overhead sunlight. It creates shadows, giving you a harsh look. Open shade is best.
3 Keep your chin up to look swan-necked and avoid the dual chin look due to the sag of age (or leftover baby fat).
4 A three-quarters shot is more flattering and more interesting than a straight-ahead pose, especially if you have a round face. Surprisingly, if your face is very narrow, three-quarters

works well too—your audience won't be sure just how much of your face is left in shadow.

5 If you have a too-prominent nose, keep your chin up a bit, and the angle of the camera will shorten it. (If you tilt your head forward or slightly downward, the camera will be focused on the broadest part of your nose.)

6 If you always wear glasses or contact lenses, keep them on for the photo. If you remove your glasses and you're very near-sighted, for example, you'll have a strange stare because you can't really see the photographer.

7 Wear your usual make-up, slightly more intensified. Just keep in mind the matte-is-best rule: You may want to use face powder even if you normally don't.

8 Don't overdo lip gloss. The wet look is not good for indoor photography because bright shine can distort the shape of lips.

9 If you have a short neck, show a little cleavage to elongate it. A too-long neck? Try a turtleneck, or cover up with an artful pose of your hands.

10 When your hands will be part of the picture, hold them up over your head first so your veins will recede (a trick I learned from hand models—it works).

11 If you have pudgy hands, hold them sideways and they'll look longer and slimmer.

12 If it's going to be a black-and-white photo, make sure the background is simple. Since everything will have the same colour value (i.e., shades of blacks and greys), if there is a tree behind you it may look like it's coming out of your ears! But don't have too much black in the background; the finished print (and you) will look muddy.

13 Even for a colour portrait, simple background is best.

14 For a colour photo, clothing in soft, feminine colours looks great. For black and white, clothes should be medium to dark to bring the face forward (grey and black are good choices).

15 Do you hate the way you smile? Learn to smile with your eyes—happy, alert eyes make the photograph come alive. Couple a slight smile with wide-awake eyes for flattering results.

MY PERSONAL PHOTOGRAPHY TIP:

o To make your face look firmer and better-shaped, with high cheekbones, put your tongue on the roof of your mouth before the pic is snapped. This pose also helps counteract an incipient double chin.

8
Nail Tech

Give me strength

There is one part of your body you can strengthen without flexing a single muscle or lifting a single weight. Unfortunately, it's not your stomach or thighs. It's your nails. No matter how weak they are, they can be toughened . . . and tougher leads to longer length.

60-SECOND NAIL HARDENER

It used to be that soft, breakable nails could be toughened only by means of commercial products containing formaldehyde (or formalin)—a known irritant. Here's my easy fast fix, and you don't need any nail tip hanging over the edge, so you can start strengthening even the shortest stubs—the harder they get, the better their chance of growing.

1 Coat the nail surface with nail glue, avoiding the cuticle.
2 Cover the nail with one coat of toilet paper. It doesn't even have to fit exactly; just leave a tiny space by the cuticle.
3 Paint over the toilet paper with glue. Let it dry completely.
4 File the surface until it's smooth. At the same time you can file away any excess toilet paper.
5 Polish your nails as usual.

THE FORMAL NAIL WRAP

To strengthen nails that peel, split or just don't seem to grow, you can try the fast fix above or go a step further and create a 'cap' to protect the edge and corners where nails tend to break. Follow this more formal wrap procedure:

1 Let your nails grow a bit. You need *some* nail to wrap—so if yours barely extend beyond your fingertips, you'll have to wait.
2 Cut your chosen paper (see next tip) in the size of a wedge that will fit over your nail. Soak the paper in the liquid provided with any nail wrapping kit and place it over the nail, including tip and corners. (If your kit tells you to buff the nail first, do so very lightly.)
3 The paper should extend slightly over the nail edge all around. Now, tuck the ends under, smoothing them into place with an

orange stick. It may help you to cut little snips along the paper edge, so you can tuck under a little bit at a time.

4 Smooth out lumps with a finger dipped in polish remover, or dip your orange stick in remover and work it over the nail. If the nail surface looks lumpy, buff it lightly to smooth it. Make sure the wrap extends underneath the nail edge; that protection is what gives the strengthening.

5 When dry, apply a coat of clear polish (making sure it extends over nail edge). Apply two coats of colour, one of sealer—and you won't need another manicure for two weeks. Your polish will stay on longer over the wraps.

6 Apply one new coat of nail enamel every night—it will protect and build strong nails along with the paper.

7 Don't be discouraged—it takes several attempts to master the technique. If you're a total failure (or just lack patience), have the job performed by a manicurist.

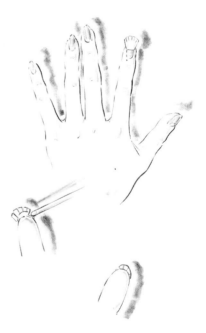

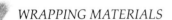 *WRAPPING MATERIALS*

While nail wrapping kits come with their own mending or wrap papers, you can customize the paper to match your manicure problem:

○ Single-ply toilet paper—the always available wrapping material.

○ Silk—for the most fragile nails. It's as thin as tissue paper, it

breathes, yet it's strong. Because it dries instantly, position silk carefully before gluing.
- Linen—another fabric, especially good for mending.
- Coffee filter or teabag paper—tried and true standbys for less fragile nails.

REMOVING NAIL WRAPS

It's not necessary! Just soak your fingertips in remover until the wrap is moist. File it down enough to smooth out the nail surface and rewrap over the old wrap. After a few manicures, if your nails are as thick as a construction worker's, you'll have to remove the whole thing.

Give me length

It doesn't take patience, just know-how to grow elegant nails fast.

THE FASTEST, EASIEST WAY TO LONG NAILS

You're in a hurry for long nails? I used to wear acrylic nails, a putty-like mix you brush on your nails in layers, using a pre-cut form to get the length and shape you want. But you do need to be something of an artist to get the natural look.

Now my fast nail hardener-plus-wrapping has given me long nails that are all mine. But you can use nail tips to achieve a long-nailed look—and there's no mixing involved. These are also good if you break a nail.

- Buy a nail tip kit in the chemist.
- Pick a plastic fake that fits your finger and glue it onto the clean nail.
- Next, glue a bit of toilet paper onto the area behind the plastic nail so your own nail and the fake are the same depth.
- Let it dry and file (where the fake and your own nail meet) until you have a smooth surface. You're ready to polish!

91

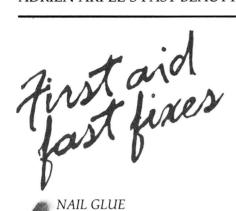

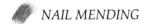 *NAIL GLUE*

While a split nail won't propel you to the head of the line in your local hospital emergency room, it is one of life's nuisances. A workable fast fix to mend the nail involves applying *one* drop of nail glue. The secret ingredient is ethyl cyanoacrylate (the same instant bonder found in many household glues). Because nail glue bonds instantly, you must use care: You don't want your fingers stuck together. And keep it far away from your eyes.

P.S.: Use nail glue specifically—it has a smaller opening than household glue, so you're less likely to apply too much and have permanently stuck-together fingers.

NAIL MENDING

○ Your nail tip is stuck in your tights? After you've finished cursing, retrieve the nail that has broken off, apply one drop of nail glue to the broken edge, and 'glue' the nail back into place. Hold the nail together until it dries.

○ Your nail broke off and you can't find it? While even perfect strangers will get down on all fours to help you search for a lost contact lens, it is socially unacceptable to ask for help in locating a lost nail. There are plastic nail tip kits available in chemists. Buy one ahead of time so you'll be ready when disaster strikes.

○ Your nail is split, but still partially attached? Cut a piece of specially designed nail mending tissue (available in nail wrapping kits), coffee filter paper or a teabag, saturate it in the mending liquid (or nail glue) and place it over the split. Cut a piece large enough to tuck in under the nail edge for added strength. Use your fingertip or orange stick to mould mending paper into position.

○ Always moisten your finger with polish remover when you work with nail mending tissues. It will help in positioning and let you smooth out the tissue more easily—you don't want a lumpy nail.

THE NUMERO UNO CAUSE OF BREAKING, SPLITTING NAILS

It's not some esoteric contaminent known only to biochemists. It's *water*. Yes, when it comes to splitting, breaking nails, H_2O is a havoc-wreaker. Keep your nails dry! Don't head for the sink without putting on cotton-lined rubber gloves—and no matter how small your hands, buy the largest size. A snug glove fit causes perspiration buildup; you're trying to avoid moisture.

SOFT, SPLITTING NAIL TIPS

○ White iodine will strengthen nails and keep them from peeling. Apply it to clean, unpolished nails every night for seven nights, then use just once a week.
○ File your nails in a squarish shape—straight across rather than oval—to resist breakage.
○ Don't go without polish. It offers a protective coat that soft nails need.
○ Bring your base coat up and around under the tip of the nail to strengthen nails and keep breakage at bay.

nail facts

Nails are made of keratin, just like hair. And, like hair too, nails are actually *dead* protein. Healthy skin around and underneath your nail promotes nail growth. Nails grow about 1/8 inch a month—a bit faster in summer than in winter. If you've lost a nail due to an accident, it will take about six months to grow back. Your middle fingernail is the fastest grower, the thumbnail the slowest. Just thought you'd like to know!

THE NAIL DIET

Since nails, like hair and skin, are protein-based, a diet rich in proteins will keep them healthy. Yes, gelatin is a protein but it will have no special effect on your nails—it's the wrong kind of protein.

NAIL 'DIAGNOSIS'

If your nails suddenly look 'sick,' separate from the nail bed, develop deep ridges, flake or become extremely brittle you may need to see the doctor. Nail health can be an indication of your overall health.

HENNA FOR NAILS

If natural (not compound) henna is an excellent hair conditioner, it follows that it is also beneficial to your nails (they're made of the same substance, remember?). Coat your fingernails in warm henna paste in a natural colour (you don't want to stain your nails and fingers) and leave on for 5 minutes. This pure, organic vegetable conditioner works for toenails, too.

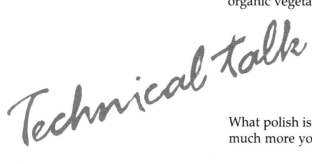

Technical talk

What polish is made of, how to store it, open it, close it . . . and much more you must know.

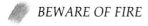

BEWARE OF FIRE

No, that's not the name of a new polish colour, it's a safety rule. Many manicure-related products (polish, remover, nail repair liquids, acrylics, et al) are highly flammable. Don't smoke or leave products near the stove or any flame when doing your nails.

FOR EASY BOTTLE OPENINGS

Rub a bit of petroleum jelly around the neck of the bottle when it's new, and it should stay easy to open for the life of the polish. If polish spills on the bottle neck, use a swab to remove it to insure a tightly closed cap. Tight closure means less air gets in, so there is less drying out and thickening.

POLISH STORAGE

Keep polish in the refrigerator. No, it doesn't grow bacteria (there's no water in it), but the cold retards thickening by stemming evaporation and polish stays liquid longer. It also arrests colour change. Before your manicure, remove polish from the refrigerator and turn the bottle upside down for half an hour, then shake gently.

Manicure memo

There's more to well-groomed hands than a slap-and-dab of polish (as you're already beginning to suspect). Here's how to insure perfection from the cuticles on up.

MANICURE STEPS: A FAST HOW-TO REVIEW

1 Remove old nail polish with cotton saturated in remover. Press the cotton onto the nail for about 15 seconds. Swish the polish off in one cuticle-to-tip stroke.
2 File the nails (make sure hands and nails are completely dry first).
3 Soak your fingers in whatever cuticle-softening liquid you prefer (hand cream, olive oil, warm sudsy water).
4 Clean your nails and fingertips with a nail brush.
5 Dry fingers, apply cuticle cream and gently push back cuticles with an orange stick wrapped in cotton or a special rubber-tipped cuticle pusher.
6 Dip the cotton-wrapped orange stick in soapy water and clean under your nails.
7 Optional: dip the stick in hydrogen peroxide to further lighten the inside of the nail tip.
8 Apply a protective, clear base coat.
9 Optional: apply nail wraps, then plastic tips.
10 Finish with two coats of your chosen colour, plus one coat of clear sealer.

PROPER FILING POSITION

Don't spread your fingers out away from you. Instead, make a fist, uncurl your fingers slightly and file with your fingers facing you. Do your thumb last. This is a comfortable working position, and it's easier to see what you're doing when your hand is curled. Always file in one direction only, using the smooth side of an emery board held under the nail at a 45-degree angle.

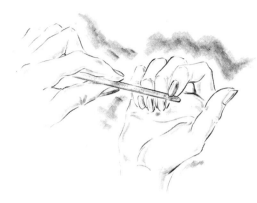

FILING SOFT, EASILY BROKEN NAILS

Leave your old polish on while filing the 'softies'. There will be less chance of nail damage. Never file nails after swimming or bathing—that's when they're at their weakest.

YELLOW NAILS TREATMENT

If you're not ill, nicotine is the probable cause. Rub half a lemon over the afflicted area. Next, remove the pulp and rub the rind vigorously over the same area to bleach it.

WARNING: A citrus-and-sunshine combo can cause permanently spotty, mottled skin, so don't apply 'lemon-aid' before you're heading for the beach or tennis courts.

REMOVING POLISH DISCOLOURATION

If your nails are stained a reddish/pinkish colour, you've been neglecting to apply base coat before polish; it's a must to prevent staining.

○ To get rid of discolouration, apply 20-volume peroxide with a cotton swab (try this method on nicotine-stained nails if the lemon rub fails).
○ Buffing helps remove stains too. Buff gently, in one direction only, from cuticle to tip. Use a buffer or the finest grade sandpaper.

NO-STREAK POLISH APPLICATION

Apply each coat of polish in three strokes. First stroke down the centre of the nail, then do either side so the side strokes meet and overlap with the centre. Don't overfill the brush; one dip into the bottle should do an entire nail.

Use the flat-out approach: The brush should be splayed out against the nail horizontally. Don't just use the tip. Flat-out means thinner layers, a more professional finish.

BUBBLY POLISH

Most common cause: polish applied to nails coated with oily residue. If you've used hand or cuticle lotion, dip a cotton swab in polish remover and whisk it over and around nails to make sure they're lotion-free.

Alternative cause: applying polish in the hot sun. Don't.

INSTANT NAIL DRYER AND SMUDGE STOPPERS

Wait 60 seconds after you apply polish and then try one of the following:

○ Apply mineral oil over the entire nail with a medicine dropper or clean brush you've saved from an old polish bottle. Set a small amount of mineral oil aside for this purpose: you don't want to contaminate your big bottle.
○ Plunge your nails into ice-cold water.
○ Buy a fast-drying nail product (either spray or liquid) from your chemist.
○ Understand that nails take about 4 hours to dry completely; these shortcuts will set polish until total drying occurs.

THE STRAIGHT-FROM-WORK MANICURE CLEAN UP

Toothpaste and a toothbrush will remove carbon and ink stains from your fingertips without ruining your manicure.

NAIL LENGTH

Don't wear your nails ridiculously long. Today's active woman will look like a useless anachronism with 'dragon lady' nails. (This advice comes from an old dragon lady—me—who has updated her look.)

Are your nails too short? Turn your palms facing you. Can't see any nails extending over your fingertips? Then your nails are too short; short nails make hands look stubby. You should see about ¼ inch of nail tip.

CHOOSING THE RIGHT NAIL SHAPE

A slightly squared oval is the most natural-looking, flattering shape. It's also a nail saver because you needn't file deeply into the sides of the nails (where most breakage starts) to achieve this shape.

CUTICLE SAVER

Soak nails in heated hand lotion to soften the cuticle before pushing back or trimming. Pushing back is preferred because the job of the cuticle is to protect the nail base (where growth occurs) from infection. Too much clipping leads to thicker, unattractive cuticles. Check out the rubber-tipped pushers in your chemist.

LET YOUR NAILS BREATHE

To insure nail growth and health, leave a smidgen of space at the base where the nail meets the cuticle (the site of regrowth) when you polish. Go bare for a few days every month.

THE FRENCH LOOK: WHITE NAIL TIPS PLUS

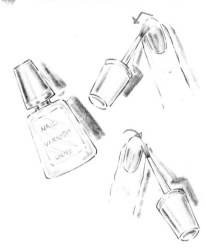

Naked-look nails are *très chic* when dressed in the French manner. This style of polishing nails was popular in the 1930s; now it's back in fashion. Try it if you have some 'tip' to your nails, and you want a polish style that will work with everything you wear.

○ Apply a base coat over the entire nail and under the tip. Let it dry.
○ Take white polish and apply it to the tip by stroking it from the outer edges to the centre on an angle.
○ Round out the bottom of the angle to a natural-looking white semicircle. Use white polish under the nail tip too. Let it dry.
○ Apply one coat of flesh-toned polish over the entire nail and under the tip.
○ Finish with a clear top coat (including the tips). You'll have beautiful, clean-looking nails, and the polish will go with everything you wear.

Colour is everything

There's no reason to lengthen and strengthen your nails if you're just going to let them hang there naked. When it comes to fingertips, colour is everything—and here is everything important you need to know about nail colour.

NAIL ENAMEL, COLOUR CUES

○ A clear, true red looks good on everyone: It's a classic colour, considered conservative because it's been in fashion for so long. Even if you can't wear red lips, your fingertips are far enough away from your face not to clash with your skin tones.

○ Stay away from browns, burgundies and maroons if your hands are starting to show signs of age, or your knuckles are big and bony.

○ If you have long, elegant fingers and well-kept nails, you can wear the deeper, more dramatic colours.

○ Nicotine-stained fingers? Wear soft pinks and shell colours. Avoid corals and tans; they'll just bring out the yellow in your fingers. This same colour rule applies if you have sallow skin.

○ If you're tanned, corals and pale frosted colours look terrific.

○ Short, stubby nails and hands look best with light or beige tones. Leave a little space on the side of each nail unpainted to make the nail look longer. Generally, the longer the nail, the brighter the colour it can take.

FROSTED, PEARLIZED POLISHES

They're terrific if you're not allergic—and today they're in fashion. But: pearlized polishes can be very 'in' one fashion season—and very 'out' the next.

MATCHING LIP AND NAIL COLOUR

No, I don't think an exact match is necessary. But you should keep the colour of your lips and nails in the same family. Light peach nail colour would look fine with coral lips; burgundy nails would not. Generally, pink, mauve or burgundy nails look best with pinky-plum lipsticks. Coral, tawny, toasty nails look best with the bronzy-toasty lip colours. True, clear reds work with both.

MATCHING CLOTHES AND NAIL COLOUR

If I am planning to wear a lot of opposing clothes colours over a week's time (between manicures), I colour my nails a flat light beige. It goes with everything.

JAZZY NAILS

For fun or special occasions, bring your manicure-one step beyond:

- Let the polish dry and apply tiny decals or stickers (or cut the decal to fit your nail).
- Use a toothpick to dot a contrasting colour over your dry polish.
- Buy glitter and dust it over wet polish.

MIX AND MATCH YOUR OWN COLOUR

I think this is an impractical waste of time, and dangerous. Polish is messy to work with, difficult to blend into good new colours—and you can blow yourself up if you're smoking.

ADD SHINE (AND COLOUR) WITHOUT POLISH

Buffing nails stimulates circulation, and it's a nice way to add shine without adding polish. You just dot on colourless or pink-tinged buffing paste, assume the same hand position as for filing, and buff gently in one direction with a special nail buffer (bought in a chemist). Fifteen seconds per nail is plenty; once a week is often enough. If you buff till your fingernails burn, you've overdone it and you're wearing down the nail.

Taking it off

Whether you've messed up your polish or are trading your red nails for pink, here are some remover fast tips I'll bet you don't know.

ABOUT POLISH REMOVER

Acetone, the key ingredient in most nail polish removers, is a drying agent, so don't think you're doing your nails a favour by removing polish daily. Instead, patch up chipped nails and do a complete new-polish manicure once a week only (or every ten days if you can stretch it).

ELIMINATING ACETONE

You probably never read the ingredients on a polish remover bottle, but all removers are *not* created equal. I've mentioned acetone removers first because they're the most common, so that's what you probably buy. Next time look for the words *butyl ethyl acetate* on the bottle. Acetates bleach and dry out the nails less than acetones.

TO REMOVE POLISH

Saturate cotton with remover, press it onto the nail, count slowly to 15, then remove fast with one swipe—this beats rubbing and gives the remover time to penetrate all the layers of polish.

Remove polish by starting at the base of the nail and working out to the tip, so you don't push the drying acetone into the delicate cuticle.

POLISH REPAIR IN A FLASH

If you mess up a nail and you're pressed for time, you don't have to take off all of the polish. Instead, dampen the pad of your opposite index finger with remover and pat the remover on the messy nail. The globby polish will smooth out sufficiently so you can let it dry and polish right over it.

REMOVER SUBSTITUTE

You have three nails left and you've run out of remover? Coat the nail with your clear base coat. Let it set for 45 seconds, press cotton over the nail and remove base plus colour in one quick swipe. It really works!

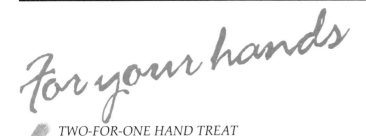

For your hands

TWO-FOR-ONE HAND TREAT

Soak your fingers in warm olive oil for a few minutes. The soak will soften cuticles and hands *and* strengthen nails.

SUPPLE HANDS WAX TREATMENT

Melt paraffin wax (found in an ironmonger) in the top of a double boiler. Apply a coat of any moisturizing cream to your hands. After testing the now-liquid wax on your inner wrist for comfortable temperature, paint it on your hands, using a narrow, clean paint brush. Let the wax harden, then remove it in large pieces, lifting dirt and debris from the skin. Rinse with cool water.

STOP CHAPPED HANDS

Leave softened lanolin on hands overnight. If your face is oily, encase your hands in cotton gloves to avoid contact and breakouts while you sleep. Your chemist should have inexpensive cotton gloves just for this purpose.

GRIT REMOVERS

Ground-in-dirt that comes from hard work when you can't wear gloves can be lifted out.

○ Wet hands in warm water and apply baby shampoo to your fingers/nails. Lather up, leave on for 1 minute, then rinse.
○ Use a pumice stone—it's not just for the feet. *Gentle* pumicing can remove roughened, dirt-filled skin.
○ Apply your mud facial mask to fingers for deep cleaning.

GRIT PREVENTER

If you have a dirty job in store, first scratch your nails several times across a wet bar of soap. Your undernails will fill up with soap, so dirt won't have room to penetrate.

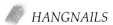 *HANGNAILS*

Keep your hands well lubricated: cracked, dry skin can lead to hangnails; so can over-exuberant cuticle trimming. Apply cuticle conditioner daily, not just during your manicure.

FOR YOUR ELBOWS

Dry, wrinkled elbows have never been considered a beauty asset, yet they're a common sight. Lubricate them every night before bed with a lanolin-rich hand cream.

Your elbows are *darker* than the rest of your arms? Rest each elbow on half a lemon for 10 minutes at a time to bleach them. In fact, take a minute out now to look at your elbows—you probably haven't done so in months, and you may be shocked.

POST-BLEACH TIP

Whenever you use lemon juice on hands or elbows (or any-where else for that matter), remember that this natural citrus bleacher is very astringent. You must follow up with a lubricating cream.

JEWELLERY, GREEN SKIN AND RASHES

Does your jewellery constantly turn your skin green? Coat the inside of your rings or bracelets with clear nail polish for anti-green protection.

Is your problem a *rash* at the jewellery site? Before you haul your jeweller into court, understand that your rash could be due to soap, water and contact dermatitis. If you keep your rings on while you wash yourself and the dishes, some of the soap or detergent will get trapped underneath, causing a breakout. Ring removal is your first step to a cure.

A Hair Care

Since I am part of a company that manages over 1100 hairdressing salons all over the world, I am in a position to show you how to make your hair stand up, lie down and roll over, curl, uncurl, unfrizz and shine, shine, shine. This chapter will give you the key to the beauty kingdom . . . beautiful hair.

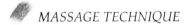

Hedonistic head ritual

There is one simple treatment you perform on your scalp that will turn you on all over: it both stimulates and relaxes, makes your whole body warm and tingly. It feels so good it almost seems it should be illegal!

MASSAGE TECHNIQUE

Theoretically, you massage your scalp to increase the circulation of blood to your head; blood carries vital nutrients to the scalp. But to hell with scientific mumbo-jumbo: it feels great.

1 Use fingertips only—not your nails, not your palms.
2 Sit in a comfortable position, bend forward, start at your collarbone, massage up to your nape.
3 Tent your fingers over the back of your scalp above the nape, underneath your hair, and massage one small area at a time using short forward-and-back strokes, then circular motions.
4 Massage until an area feels tingly and warm, then move on.
5 Do the back of the head first, work to the sides and front, finish with the crown. Follow with shampoo.

LUBRICATE FIRST

To increase your pleasure and make finger movements easier, moisten your scalp with the appropriate lotions. Choose what's right for you, section hair in 1-inch widths and dampen the scalp at each parting with a saturated cotton ball. Rewet your fingers in solution as necessary. (You follow a massage with shampoo, so don't worry about the mess.)

Dry, tight scalp? Warm some olive oil and mix in 1 teaspoon wheat germ oil, ½ teaspoon oil of rosemary, 3 drops of lavender oil.

Oily scalp? Mix 3 ounces of witch hazel, 3 ounces of mineral water and the pulp of 1 lemon.

Normal scalp? Make a mixture that is ½ rosewater, ½ mineral water and add 1 teaspoon of cologne.

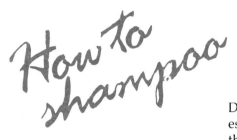

Did you know that many hair problems are due to nothing more esoteric than botched hair washing efforts? Make sure you're in the minority who shampoo right.

HAIR WASHING WATER TEMPERATURE

Hair can't stand excruciating heat, whether it's in the form of blow-drying or very hot water. Wash your hair in warm water, but finish up with an ice-cold rinse. Here's the cold rationale: shampoo swells and raises the cuticle—that's how it gets in to clean. But light only reflects off a smooth, flat surface. So if you want reflected light (i.e., shine) on your hair, the cuticle must be flat and closed. Cold water closes the cuticle and promotes healthy shine.

HOW TO SHAMPOO

1 Always brush your hair before shampooing to get oil away from scalp. This will make washing easier; you won't have to scrub so hard.
2 Make sure your hair is thoroughly combed, hanging loose down your back. Don't pile it up in one place. Let the water run over your hair for 60 seconds.
3 Pour shampoo into the palm of your hand and mix it with a bit of water before applying to your head.
4 Run shampoo-coated fingers and palms through loose wet hair. This distributes the cleanser better, and you will use less shampoo and create lather. The less you use, the easier it is to remove every last drop.
5 Massage with your fingertips, concentrating on scalp and areas close to roots. The ends are usually dryer and cleaner because scalp oils don't reach that far. Three minutes is long enough.
6 Rinse. See page 00 for how-tos.

DAILY DOSES

If you wash your hair every day, 1 teaspoon (2 teaspoons for long hair) of shampoo will suffice; if you use more, you're engaging in hard-to-rinse-out overkill. Lather only once.

THE SKIN/SCALP CONNECTION

You're not sure if you have an oily or a dry scalp? Hint: if your face is oily, so is your scalp. That's a rule of nature. Your hair may be dry due to perming, colouring, mechanical abuse—but don't trick yourself into thinking that any scalp topping a face with oily skin is dry. It doesn't work that way.

THE SKIN/SCALP CONNECTION, PART II

If your oily scalp is combined with dry hair (due to perms, colouring, daily blow-drying, etc.), how can you wash your scalp often enough without your hair turning to straw? Simple: wet hair and add conditioners first. This will protect your hair while you shampoo your scalp with gusto (of course, conditioners don't go near the scalp).

THE DAILY SHAMPOO SCALP OIL MYTH

It's not daily washing that causes the scalp's oil glands to work overtime—it's washing with too-harsh shampoos that strip the hair of natural oil so the scalp is forced to overcompensate.

SHAMPOO SELECTION

Unfortunately, it's largely a matter of trial and error, with your mirror being the final judge. Omit some errors by matching labels to your hair condition (i.e., for dry, oily, colour-treated or blow-dried hair). It also helps to ask your stylist for a recommendation.

SHAMPOO TIP FOR THE SUPER OILY

No matter how frequently you wash, your hair still looks greasy? Next time, apply your diluted shampoo to dry hair and start working up a little lather. Since oil and water don't mix, wetting your hair thoroughly first may not be the answer. Once you've worked the shampoo in, wet and wash as usual.

THE BIG (SHAMPOO) SWITCH

You needn't be a dandruff sufferer to benefit from alternating shampoos. Find a few you like, and switch between them. Shampoos have many different ingredients, and your hair will benefit from the cornucopia of cleansers and additives. (And, yes, hair does stop responding to the same old thing after a while—switching products puts off that problem.)

WHAT ABOUT BABY SHAMPOOS?

Leave them to baby; they don't clean adult hair thoroughly. Here's why: hair has a negative charge. Sebum, grease, hair spray, dirt, conditioners and the like are positively charged. Because positives and negatives attract, hair 'garbage' clings to hair. The typically *anionic* shampoo of adults is negatively charged, so it releases positively charged scalp debris.

Now (hang on, I'm almost finished!) baby shampoo is *amphoteric*, which means it has both positive and negative charges; to clean your hair you must accentuate the negative—and since baby shampoos don't do that, they're weak cleansers.

The rinse factor

What you take out of your hair is much more important than what you put in. That's why thorough rinsing is so critical. It's the only way to get rid of shampoo, extra conditioners, etc. Poor rinsing guarantees dull, greasy hair. Besides rinsing *out* debris, you can rinse *in* beauty. What follows is a rinse roundup.

RINSING LONG OR THICK HAIR

You can't just direct the spray to the top of your hair and expect the water to seep through and do a thorough cleansing job. Instead, lift your hair and rinse one section at a time. Then lean forward and rinse the whole mass.

AFTER-SHAMPOO RESIDUE REMOVERS

What if you never feel you've removed all traces of shampoo, no matter how long you rinse? This problem is especially difficult if you're in a hard-water area. You need an acidic rinse to get rid of the anionic shampoo and help flatten your cuticles and encourage shine.

○ For dark hair, mix 1 part apple cider vinegar to 4 parts water, and add 5 drops oil of cloves.
○ For blonde hair, use 1 part lemon juice and 4 parts water.
○ Pour the mixture over your shampooed, rinsed hair as a final rinse. Leave it in.

WARNING: Don't pour straight vinegar onto your hair. It will strip the hair of essential oils.

LEMON JUICE SIDE EFFECT

While it makes a nice brightening and acidic rinse, lemon juice can also be drying. Make sure you condition hair regularly if you're a juice fan.

SHINE-IN RINSE

If your dark hair is dull and tends to be oily, take 3 tablespoons of rosemary and 2 tablespoons of sage. Boil them in 3 pints of water for 15 minutes. Strain, let it come to room temperature and refrigerate. Pour this over your hair and let it sit for 2 minutes. Rinse. You should notice a nice shine.

RINSES THAT ADD ZING TO NATURAL HAIR COLOUR

○ Blondes: brew a cup of camomile tea; strain.
○ Brunettes: brew a cup of espresso.
○ Redheads: brew a cup of Orange tea, or dilute beet juice; strain.

Shampoo, pour the *cooled* liquid through your hair, let it sit for 5 minutes; rinse well.

CREAM RINSE SUBSTITUTE

A teaspoon of liquid fabric softener stirred into 1 cup of warm water and poured over your head works in an emergency if you're out of cream rinse and need help untangling your hair.

Conditioning cues

Your hair probably needs extra help. That's what conditioners provide. Even if your hair is in good shape, it needs at least an occasional conditioning to stay that way because every time you wash your hair you open and swell the cuticle—and conditioners close the cuticle, promoting shine as well as health. The conditioners also restore needed moisture and protein to the hair shaft, not necessarily oil. If you have oily hair, look for an *oil-free* conditioner.

CONDITION WITH CONFIDENCE

If your conditioner leaves your hair with a heavy, lank feeling, your major mistake is that you're probably following directions! All conditioners, regardless of label instructions, should be diluted with water.

Apply the conditioner with a 1-inch paint brush or your fingers, starting an inch from the scalp. Run your fingers through the hair to distribute the conditioner. Don't touch your scalp with conditioner—it's for hair only. And don't massage in a conditioner—it just coats the hair.

The most conditioning should be devoted to the bottom half of your hair and the ends: because this is the oldest section of your hair, it's had the most abuse and needs the most help.

KEEP YOUR CONDITIONER FROM DISINTEGRATING

Too much heat can break down your conditioner. Here's what happens: if you hold your hair dryer too close to your newly conditioned head, the heat will melt the conditioner and it won't be able to do its job. While warmth activates it, too-hot heat destroys conditioner.

CONDITIONING FOR THE OIL-PRONE

You have a terribly oily scalp but your hair still needs conditioning? With everything we do to our hair (blow-drying, perming, colouring, exposing it to pollutants), most of us need to condition every time we wash. The trick: condition hair before you shampoo, rather than the other way around. Wet your hair, towel it dry, and apply your favourite conditioner starting an inch away from your scalp. Work the conditioner through your hair, wait and rinse. Now, shampoo as usual.

NOTE: Fine hair that tends to go limp when conditioned can also benefit from conditioners if you follow this condition-first shampoo-last technique.

BOOST YOUR DEEP CONDITIONER

If you're giving yourself an intensive 30-minute conditioning treatment, give it a boost by mixing in 1 teaspoon of vitamin E oil.

CONDITIONER ANTIDOTE

While conditioner works to strengthen your hair, it can leave a dulling coat if not rinsed out thoroughly. Here is a super conditioner rinse-out to make at home. Keep it in the shower in a large plastic bottle.

For dark hair, use 4 tablespoons of rosemary; for light hair, 4 tablespoons of camomile. Boil 4 cups of water and pour it over your chosen herb. Let it cool.

When applying, bring a nonbreakable bowl or pot into the shower. Bend over, pour the herbed water over your head and catch the fallout in pot. Reapply to your hair as often as you have liquid left.

Dry shampoo

WHEN YOU CAN'T SHAMPOO

You don't even have time for a dry cleaning? At least your hair will smell fresh if you put astringent or cologne on a cotton ball and dab it all around your hairline from the nape to the crown. This is an especially effective hot-weather cooler.

RESIDUE-FREE DRY CLEANING FOR HAIR

Sprinkle a piece of cheesecloth with cologne, cover a brush with it and brush your hair thoroughly. Your hair will smell as well as look cleaner.

BRUSHING AWAY DIRT

When you're too sick to wash your hair (but looking at your greasy head makes you sicker), you need a dry shampoo.

Put either cornflour or cornmeal in a spice jar with large holes (so you won't dump out too much at once) and sprinkle lightly over your head. Now, push a piece of lightly woven cotton, cheesecloth, tights or (if your dirt is upscale!) silk through the bristles of your hairbrush. The powder will dislodge the debris; the cloth will trap excess grease.

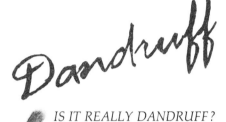

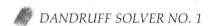

IS IT REALLY DANDRUFF?

Lightly flaking scalp could be due to shampoo residue or left-over hair spray, or it could be a more serious seborrhea condition that should be seen by a dermatologist. Self-test; skip setting lotions, mousses, gels, sprays, conditioners for two weeks. Rinse away your shampoo three times as long as usual. Try parting the hair and giving your scalp a warm olive oil treatment if your scalp feels dry (see page 113). Do this twice a week for one week.

If your flaking is due to an oily scalp, try Dandruff Solver No. 1 or 2 below. If these treatments don't work, try the commercial shampoos featuring tar and other special ingredients.

Still no relief? Now it's time for a dermatologist.

DANDRUFF SOLVER NO. 1

Dandruff occurs when the normal process of skin shedding speeds up, goes haywire, and large stuck-together scales peel off en masse. Before you use an anti-dandruff shampoo, use an antiseptic to clean up your oily scalp (most dandruff is caused by too much, not too little, oil. Dilute 1 part mouthwash (use yellowy or clear brands rather than red or green ones) to 4 parts water. If that's not effective, work up to ½ antiseptic, ½ water. Part your hair in 1-inch sections and apply the solution with a saturated cotton ball. Leave it on for 1 hour or overnight, covering your hair with a shower cap. Just shampoo when you're finished.

DANDRUFF SOLVER NO. 2

Mix 2 tablespoons of any 'colourless' mouthwash with 2 tablespoons of witch hazel and 4 tablespoons of mineral water. Add a few drops of cologne for fragrance. Apply by parting your hair in 1-inch sections with the handle of a fine paint brush, and paint the mix on your scalp with the brush proper.

MOISTURIZING SCALP TREATMENT

If you suspect your flaking scalp is due to dryness, mix 2 ounces of glycerin with ½ ounce of apple cider vinegar. Section your hair and apply the mixture with cotton balls. Leave it on for 15 minutes, then rinse.

NOTE: This also helps heal a sunburned scalp.

FAST ANTI-DANDRUFF LOTION

After you wash your hair and before you dry it, saturate a cotton ball with witch hazel and apply it to your scalp at ½-inch intervals.

COMMERCIAL DANDRUFF ZAPPERS

If you have dandruff, you must study shampoo labels. The ingredients that work are sulphur, zinc, tar, salycylic acid and selenium pyrithicone. Buy a couple of dandruff shampoos containing different variations of the above ingredients to determine which works best for you. If you've tried the do-it-yourself tips I've suggested and dandruff shampoos and you still get no relief, see a dermatologist.

NOTE: Dandruff shampoos are not terribly gentle; they're not the best thing for permed or coloured hair.

Special treats

If your hair hangs out in all kinds of weather, in all the wrong places, it deserves an occasional boost.

OLIVE OIL

This is the best all-around conditioner ever discovered for dry, damaged hair. You can even use it on tinted hair without fear. Proceed as follows:

1 Heat olive oil until it's warm, not hot.
2 Section your hair at ½-inch intervals and apply the oil to partings with a pastry or paint brush.
3 Comb your hair with a wide-toothed rubber comb to distribute oil from the scalp to ends.
4 When hair and scalp are saturated (apply only to hair if scalp is oily), cover your head with plastic wrap, and around it all wrap a towel saturated in hot water and wrung out. Heat helps penetration.
5 Leave on 15 minutes.
6 To remove, apply shampoo to your head, massage it in and then add water. (Remember, oil and water don't mix.) Lather twice and work the shampoo in well. Rinse—rinse—rinse!

OLIVE OIL SUBSTITUTE

Try coconut oil or sesame oil if you hate all the scrubbing necessary to remove olive oil.

TWO HIGH PER TREATMENTS

PER = Protein Efficiency Ratio, and two hair helpers that have it are soy sauce and whey.

Soy sauce is 50 percent hydrolized vegetable protein, excellent for hair. Stir 1 ounce of sauce into 1 cup of warm water. Pour this over your hair after shampooing. Rinse it out after 10 minutes.

Whey is another protein-enricher. Use 1 ounce per 1 cup of warm water and pour it through your hair after shampooing. Leave it on for 10 minutes, then rinse. To retrieve whey from cottage cheese, see page 11.

ALL-NIGHTER FOR TERMINALLY DRY HAIR

If your hair is extremely dry and damaged, leave your 10-minute deep conditioning treatment on overnight, wrapping your hair in plastic.

'CHOLESTEROL' HAIR TREATMENT

While egg yolks may be bad for your heart, they're great for your hair. Combine 2 egg yolks, ½ teaspoon of shampoo, 1 cup warm (not hot) water. Beat it all together. Apply this to your wet hair, massage it in, leave on for 5 minutes and rinse.

HAIR RESTORER

Mix soya oil and the pulp of an avocado until you have a thin paste. If you have a dry scalp as well as dry hair, apply the mixture to both. If your scalp is oily and your hair is dry, apply paste at least 1 inch away from your scalp.

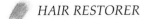

Nutrients

Your hair, like your body, reflects what you consume. Here are some thoughts on conspicuously healthy consumption.

WHAT TO FEED YOUR HAIR

It's not enough to coat hair with conditioners; you must also nourish it—and hair, made from a protein called keratin, loves protein to the tune of 50 to 60 grams a day. Your diet should be rich in liver, fish, veal, eggs, chicken, turkey or lowfat milk and cheese.

NOTE: One tablespoon of cold-pressed oil (the unprocessed variety of oil found in health food stores) added to your daily diet will help lubricate dry hair.

VITAMINS FOR THE HAIR

There's a whole alphabet soup of vitamins and minerals that are really wonder drugs for the hair:

○ B complex vitamins not only strengthen the hair shaft, they promote hair growth. One B complex capsule daily will help. Brewer's yeast and dessicated liver are excellent dietary B sources.

○ The Anti-B's: caffeine, sugar, starches and alcohol are B drainers. Avoid them. The Pill also has an adverse effect on vitamin B; make sure there's a B complex in your diet if you take the Pill.

○ The scalp circulation-boosting vitamin is E. Start with 100 units a day; top off at 400. Wheat germ oil, nuts and grains are E-rich; the Pill is an E-robber.

NOTE: If you have high blood pressure or circulatory problems, don't take E without a doctor's approval.

○ Vitamin C helps rebuild key hair production tissues and it encourages good circulation (important because blood carries nutrients to your scalp). Stress, smoking and aspirin are C robbers; 1000 mg of vitamin C per day (half in the morning, half at night) is a good hair-helping amount.

MINERALS FOR THE HAIR

○ Iron is essential, but don't prescribe for yourself—let your doctor test you and prescribe iron supplements if necessary.
○ If you're cursed by weak hair and fallout, zinc may help. Take it as part of a multimineral supplement or find it in food form: spinach, shellfish, sunflower seeds.
○ Copper fights grey hair. Find it in nuts and raisins. (Caution: Does your drinking water flow through copper pipes? You may be getting more than enough.)

NOTE: Always take these minerals and any others as part of a balanced multimineral supplement. Don't try to calculate dosage on your own.

Hair Health

Is yours in good shape? Are you losing it? Read on.

THE BOUNCE-BACK HAIR HEALTH TEST

Not sure about the state of your hair? Remove one strand from the front of your head near the crown; gently stretch it. If it's healthy, it should stretch 20 to 25 percent of its normal length, then bounce back. Dry, damaged hair will break before it stretches to the desired length.

BROKEN VS. BALDING

When there's an unusually large handful of hair on your brush or pillow, you'll want to determine if the hair has broken off due to mishandling (overprocessing, too much perming, bleaching, blow-drying or too many ponytails) or, more seriously, if it's coming out at the scalp. Hold the hair up to a magnifying mirror: Do you see a bit of white at the root? That means your hair is coming out rather than breaking off—a time-for-the-dermatologist problem. If you're not sure, and you're unhappy with the amount of hair strewn about the house, see one anyway.

Exercise

SWEAT AND HAIR

If you work up a sweat, you can use your aerobic dancing, running or tennis time to tune up your hair as well as your body. Comb conditioner through your hair, cover it with a hat and work out. The heat and sweat from your scalp will activate the conditioner and give you a good 30- to 60-minute deep penetrating conditioning. Shampoo as soon as you're finished.

The sweat on your scalp contains salt, which is drying. So even if you don't condition, you must shampoo after exercise.

AFTER-SPORTS HAIR LIVENER

Mix your shampoo dose with 1 cup of Perrier water for a light cleanser that feels wonderfully active and alive. Experiment: you will be able to use less shampoo than usual because the bubbly Perrier will create lots of lather.

Styling options

MOST OVERLOOKED STYLING TOOL . . .

Your fingers! They won't do damage. Run them through your hair. Scrunch and fluff hair up. Finger-dry after you towel-dry and eliminate the need for some blow-drying and setting.

MOUSSE VS. GEL VS. SETTING LOTION

When to use what? Use a fluffy mousse when you want a defined, spiky style that needs lots of separation and hold. Gels or glazes give a sleek, full or wet look. Setting lotions impart control and body when you're setting your hair with rollers or hot rollers. By the way, you can control the strength of your setting lotion by diluting it with water.

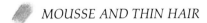 ## MOUSSE AND THIN HAIR

If you have thin hair, plopping on a mousse can weight it down, making it look thinner and greasy. Here's a great tip to help you get the mousse benefits: part your hair in 1-inch sections and spray hair spray along the part lines. Let it dry completely. Now, apply just a touch of mousse and you'll have soft control without sacrificing body.

TWO QUICK TWISTS ON ROLLERS

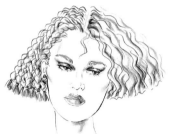

○ Twist Fix No. 1: if you can't stand rollers, but would like an occasional curl, use pipecleaners. You can easily wind damp hair around them for tight no-pins/no-fuss curls.
○ Twist Fix No. 2: plait your hair. The skinnier the plait, the tighter the curl; thicker plaits make larger waves. BONUS: You can leave the house wearing plaits, while setting foot in public with a head full of curlers is cause for arrest.

STYLING REMINDERS

Some styles last only a season; others, with variations, go on forever. Whether you prefer the trendy or the classic, here are some thoughts to keep in mind before your next salon visit:

○ Don't leave the hairdresser's looking like a pinhead. If you're very tall, a very short haircut won't be flattering.
○ If you're short, don't overpower your face and body with too much long, full hair.
○ If you're chubby-faced, consider a style that waves around your jawline rather than a severe pulled-back look.
○ Fringes camouflage a too-high or too-broad forehead and draw attention to marvellous eyes.

TO TRIM YOUR FRINGE

Nothing is as foolproof as going to a salon, but if you want to try it on your own:

○ Schedule your trim for after your shampoo. Hair must be clean and wet for accurate results.

○ Clip all non-fringe hair out of the way.
○ Comb fringe hair forward and clamp it down flat with hair-setting tape no more than ¼ inch from the ends.
○ Wet your hair again if it's starting to dry.
○ Start with the centre section right above your nose.
○ Your first snip shouldn't be shorter than below the eyebrows. Keep snipping all the way to the right; return to the centre cut and move all the way to the left.
○ Never try to remove more than ¼ inch (preferably ⅛ inch) at a time.

KEEP FRINGE FROM DRYING CURLY

Apply hair-setting tape to your fringe when it's wet, approximately ¼ inch from edge. Blow-dry.

TO CONTROL UNRULY CURLY HAIR . . .

Get a layered haircut. That way the curls won't be long enough to go every which way.

BROKEN ENDS 'CURE'

You've tried every conditioner on earth? Get a haircut. It works every time. If you don't remove broken ends, they will continue to split up the shaft.

CONTROL FRIZZY TROPICAL HAIR

If you have wavy hair, have it cut all one length. It will appear straight and be easier to blow straight. When you take wavy hair to a humid tropical paradise, be prepared to look like you just stuck your whole head in a socket. Solution: pair your electrified hair with funky clothes and everyone will think that's the look you worked hours to achieve.

FIGHT FRIZZY ENDS

If it's just your ends that curl and crinkle, coat them with a bit of olive oil before setting or blow-drying for increased manageability. P.S.: a dab of olive oil goes a long way.

GROWING LONG HAIR

If you do want to let your hair grow, whether you're letting a layered look grow out or just want l-o-n-g hair, save your trims for the cold weather. Heat seems to stimulate hair growth, so if you leave your hair alone during the summer, you'll take full advantage of this seasonal growth spurt.

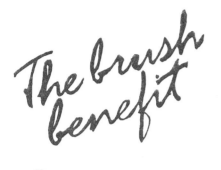

Brushing can cleanse and impart fullness, or it can destroy your hair. Make sure your technique is on the side of the angels.

BRUSH AND COMB TYPING

The finer your hair, the softer the bristles should be. Natural hair bristles are best for everyone, but if your hair is so ultra-thick you can barely get a brush through, look for a natural bristle and nylon combination. Buy a wide-toothed comb of rubber or real tortoiseshell only. Skip plastic and metal.

BRUSHING HOW-TOS

- Use a comb to untangle dry hair first.
- Make sure your brush touches your scalp. The purpose of brushing is to distribute the oils from the scalp along the hair shaft to the ends of your hair.
- If you have dry hair, you should brush more frequently than if you have oily hair. But in any case, 15 to 50 strokes is enough.
- When you brush, bend over from the waist and let hair fall over your eyes; this is the most efficient position for getting out dirt, distributing oil, imparting fullness.
- To brush for fullness, start bent over, stroking from nape area. Brush from the roots to the ends. Now, toss your head back and smooth the hair slightly with your fingertips.

BRUSH CLEANSING

Here's a fast fix for grimy hairbrushes that works every time. Make a mix of 2 tablespoons of baking soda, 2 tablespoons of colourless mouthwash and enough water to cover the hairbrush. Wash the brush for 15 minutes. Rinse it thoroughly in clear water and blow-dry it. If you want it to self-dry, lay the brush bristles down on a towel.

NOTE NO. 1: Why baking soda? Detergent soaps will soften bristles.

NOTE NO. 2: Plastic brushes and handles can be submerged and left. Keep a wooden handle out of the water and just swirl the bristles through it.

NOTE NO. 3: While a good soaking is necessary, so is some manual labour. Take a clean eyebrow brush or a child's toothbrush and scrub between and around the rows of bristles.

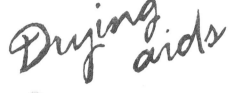

BLOW-DRYING RULES

○ 1000 watts should be the maximum heat you use.
○ Don't use your blow-dryer on completely dry hair (it's not that kind of styling tool); you'll damage your hair.
○ Don't use your blower on completely wet hair; you'll need too much heat for too long and you'll encourage broken ends. Towel-dry and finger-dry your hair as much as possible before you begin. Let hair air-dry as long as possible.
○ Use higher heat until hair is at least halfway dry, switch to a lower setting.
○ Start at the nape and work forward. Do the delicate crown and sides last.
○ For fullness, assume the same bent over, all-hair-forward position you use for brushing.

FAST FIX FOR OILY HAIR

You just washed and dried your hair and it's oily already? Don't necessarily blame your shampoo—that gushing scalp could be due to a faulty drying technique. For oily heads, set that blow-dryer only on LOW. High settings stimulate the scalp's oil production mechanism.

HOW TO AVOID KINKY HAIR

If you never seem to get that smooth look you're aiming for, you're probably leaving your under-hair (especially the section at the nape of the neck) damp. Bend forward and brush all hair upside down over your face, then blow-dry for a sleeker look.

BEST DRYING TOOL FOR CURLY HAIR.

Mother Nature. If you have no time to wait, invest in an infra-red heat bulb. It dries your hair without any blowing or touching, so the curl doesn't get mechanically smashed and bashed. Ask the professionals at your salon where they get theirs.

HOW TO TELL IF YOUR ELECTRIC ROLLERS ARE TOO HOT

Simple: give a feel. Does your finger burn? So will your hair. Use only a steam-producing variety. To avoid split ends, wrap hair in end papers before rolling.

BLOW-DRYING AND STATIC ELECTRICITY

They seem to go together. As you dry, run the palm of your free hand over your hair. It will keep the flyaways calm. When you're finished, take a drop of hand cream, rub well into your palms and run them over your finished style for a stay-in-place finishing touch.

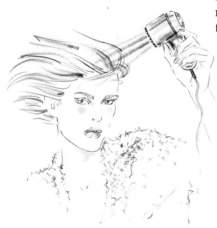

TAMING STATIC ELECTRICITY

Apply a coat of hairspray to the inside of your palm and after each brush stroke run your open palm over your hair. Reapply spray to your hand as often as necessary.

TIP FOR WINTER SHOCK

Hair tends to stand straight up in winter (due to the static electricity caused by central heating). To cope: spray your hairbrush with hairspray and brush it gently over your hair.

Colouring: the most fabulous fast fix

Colour can cause the most awful hair problems if used incorrectly. But when it's done right? Spectacular, a makeover in itself! Here are important things to know and do before you take the plunge.

DETERMINING YOUR NATURAL HAIR COLOUR

If you've permed, used colour in the past, or if you dry your hair with heat or sit in the sun often, it's not that easy to determine this.

○ First, follow the artists' lead and go to a north-facing window with your mirror; north offers 'true light'. Studying your hair under fluorescents won't give you a true reading. Always test in daylight.

○ Make sure your hair is clean and dry. Dirty, oily, wet hair distorts the colour.

○ The colour you see head-on has been affected by all the processing and daily trauma you (and I) subject your hair to. Check the colour of your hair near your scalp—it's the newest hair not yet affected by mechanical manipulation, chemicals or sun.

○ To decide what hair colour you want, take a strand from the back of the head (it's darkest there) *and* a strand from the front hairline (lightest). Decide which shade you like, but remember that people most often see you head-on—the angle at which your hair is naturally lightest.

FAST FACTS TO AVOID GARISH HAIR COLOUR MISTAKES

○ You want to duplicate the colour on the package exactly? Forget it. The model's hair was probably bleached completely white before the colouring job.

○ Consider the harsh reality of the genetic code. You really do look best if you don't flaunt Mother Nature. If you have olive skin and dark eyes, you will look strange as a light blonde. If you were born with very fair skin, and are blonde, you will look like you're ready for Halloween if you go black. But do consider going one or two shades lighter or darker, and adding subtle highlights or streaking.

○ If you can sneak into a wig department and try on a few in different shades, you'll see what I mean about not straying too far from your natural colour.

○ Considering trading in your grey hair for the colour of your youth? Don't aim for an exact return to yesteryear. As you age (and in hair terms the changes can start at thirty-five or younger), your hair fades—it starts to turn white. Well, your skin also gets a shade or two lighter. If you go for the dark hair you had at sixteen, your face may look too ghastly pale by contrast.

QUICK COLOUR CHART FOR THE NOVICE

Just to make sure you and the colourist speak the same language (or you're buying the right kit if you plan to go it alone), study the following:

TYPE	LASTS	CONTAINS PEROXIDE	EFFECTS
Temporary rinse	1 shampoo	No	Highlights; provides subtle shade uplifts; can wash out in rain.
Semi-permanent rinse	4–6 shampoos	No	Creates highlights; enhances grey; covers grey without changing the rest of your hair. Good for experimenting.
Henna	Until you cut it off	No (its a vegetable dye)	Adds dramatic highlights and colour; can be unpredictable; fades gradually all over so no root retouch is necessary.

TYPE	LASTS	CONTAINS PEROXIDE	EFFECTS
Permanent aniline-derivative tints			
1) One-step	Until you cut it off	Yes	Hair is both lightened and coloured in one step because peroxide is mixed right in with tint. You can go several shades darker or lighter than natural colour; covers grey. Roots must be retouched.
2) Double process	Until you cut it off	Yes	Bleaching is done in a separate step to strip hair of colour. Used to turn hair from dark brown to very blonde. Retouching a must. Hard on hair.

PATCH TESTS ARE FOR EVERYONE

Before each application (even a product you've used before—you never know when an allergy may develop), patch-test for safety and strand-test for satisfactory results. To strand-test, take a small bit of hair and preview the colour before doing your whole head.

HELP FOR THE ALLERGY-PRONE

If your test shows you're allergic or sensitive to the formula, patch-test using frosting or streaking techniques. With these methods chemicals don't (they shouldn't!) touch the scalp, so you *may* be able to use some colour after all.

THE COLOUR CURE FOR THIN, LIMP HAIR

You think fine hair should be left alone? Wrong! If it's healthy, colouring can give fine hair body and bounce. Here's why: permanent colouring opens the cuticle so hair colour can penetrate the inner layer of the hair shaft. Once the shaft has swollen to accommodate the colour, it reseals. The result: a fatter shaft, thicker hair.

AVOID KINKY GREYS

If you start to go grey early, blame it on heredity, but don't get so upset that you pull your greys out one hair at a time. They'll still grow back grey! Worse, the greys thus removed will be replaced by coarser, slightly coiled strands. Leave them alone and at least they'll match the growth pattern and texture (if not the colour) of the rest of your hair.

FAST FIX FOR 'GREEN' HAIR

Bleach and chlorine are a disastrous combination. If your hair turns green after a day at the pool, shame on you! Don't swim without wearing a cap or at least coating your hair with conditioner. Remedy: Dissolve 6 to 8 aspirins (depending on hair length) in warm (not hot) water. Pour this over your head. Let it sit for 10–15 minutes and rinse. Most of the green should disappear.

HOW TO KILL YOUR HAIR

Never perm and colour hair on the same day. If you want to do both, perm first and colour 10 days later. But please, no double-process blonding and perming! That's one chemical step too many for hair.

STREAKING AND SUCH

If you're considering streaking, you're onto a good thing:

○ Streaking, frosting and hair painting are relatively untraumatic. The alkaline chemicals don't touch your scalp, and not all your hair is subjected to the processing.
○ You can wait up to 6 months for a retouch, because the colour is shot all through your hair without touching the root line.

CHEATING AT RETOUCHING

Get rid of your parting. The roots along your parting will be highly visible, even across a crowded room. If you have a curly, no-parting style, you can wait longer between touch-ups.

TINTED HAIR CARE PRIMER

○ Shampoo less frequently—your hair may feel dryer due to oxidation. Lather only once.
○ Use an instant 60-second conditioner every time you wash your hair.
○ Keep tinted hair out of the sun. Don't swim in chlorine without first applying a conditioner or putting on a cap.
○ Give yourself a monthly warm olive oil treatment.

ABOUT HENNA

Consider it if you want dramatic colour that fades all over, eliminating frequent root retouches. But understand that the results are unpredictable. For big colour changes, use traditional colouring agents. Also the henna-and-water paste mix you plop on your head is messy to use.

Never henna over permed or coloured hair. And *never* perm or colour over henna. Which means once you've done it, you must live with your new look until it fades or you cut it off.

TAKING HENNA ONE STEP BEYOND

Once you've had some experience with henna paste, jazz it up:

○ For body and shine without noticeable colour change, add 1 egg to natural henna.
○ For slight blonding, add lemon juice to a light brown henna.
○ To dramatize black henna still further, substitute espresso coffee for the plain hot water.
○ To give dark brown hair even greater red highlights, substitute tea for the necessary water.
○ To tone down auburn highlights, substitute tea for the necessary water.
○ Spice it up. A dash of red pepper is said to impart a bright auburn glow; ginger lends red highlights to brown henna. Add spice directly to the powder.

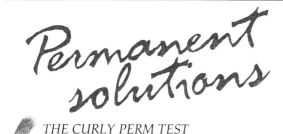

Permanent solutions

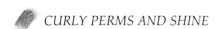 *THE CURLY PERM TEST*

You're not sure how you'll look with a curly perm? Give yourself a preview, and avoid months of living with an I-hate-curly-hair disaster. Next time you shampoo, plait your wet hair into as many small plaits as you can (it helps to have a friend do the back for you). Let your hair dry completely without benefit of a blow-dryer. (This could take several hours.) Now, carefully unwind the plaits, shake your head and study yourself in the mirror. If you like what you see, you're ready for a perm.

CURLY PERMS AND SHINE

Sorry, it's difficult to have both.

First, the alkaline chemicals used in processing raise the cuticle, the hair's outer cover, which must be flat for lots of shine.

Second, blame the curls themselves. Light is reflected off flat surfaces, and your curls are not lying against the side of your head, so light can't reflect off them properly.

Third, you don't brush your perm from scalp to ends (you gently lift with a pick), so the scalp oils never get distributed through your hair and it stays dry looking.

To compensate:

○ Don't lather more than once, and don't shampoo daily. Even if your pre-permed locks were oily, processing has dried them out somewhat, and too much stripping will remove essential oils further.

○ Brushing is a curl-destroyer, but you can engage in vigorous scalp massage to make sure those oils don't stay completely scalp-locked.

○ Don't shampoo without applying a 60-second protein-rich conditioner to help close your swollen, cracked cuticle.

○ Fake a shine by rubbing a dab of petroleum jelly, gel or mousse through your hair.

○ To revive a curly perm, just fill a plant sprayer with cold water and spray it over your hair. It's the simplest pick-me-up between shampoos.

Jazz it up

USING DECORATIVE HAIR COMBS

If yours fall out, consider:

Matching the comb type to your hair type. If you have short hair, you need a comb with short teeth; long hair needs a comb with longer teeth.

Calculate the amount of hair you want to 'catch' and match the comb width to the look you're aiming for.

Slick a thin layer of setting gel over the area of the hair where you'll be inserting the comb. It should keep it in place.

To insure that the comb will stay put, first direct the teeth in the opposite direction from the way you want it to sit, then turn the comb back to reweave through the same hair.

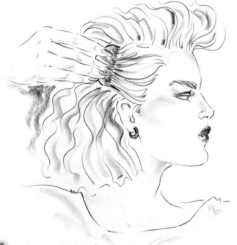
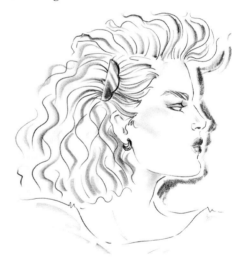

NIGHT LIGHTS

○ Gold streaks: Mist hairspray over one section of your hair; dust on gold (or silver, pink—whatever strikes your fancy) glitter. The spray will keep glitter in place.
○ Don't like hairspray? Dust glitter over setting gel.
○ Hate the look and tightness of rubber bands? Finish off your plait with a large costume jewellery ring.
○ Entwine a rope of pearls or other beads in your hair.
○ Use clip-on earrings as hair accessories.
○ Remember silk flowers and feathers.

10
Sun
Worshipping

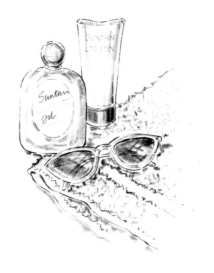

For an ear of corn ripening on the stalk, the sun is the giver of life. For a woman who'd rather stay ripe than wizened, an intelligent approach to the sun is in order.

Here's everything you need to know about protection, sun and acne, sun and hair colour, faking a tan and the (very few) good uses for the sun.

Don't leave for vacation without reading this chapter!

Your most critical decision

To insure a burn-free summer that won't promote skin aging, your number one decision won't be whether to head for the beach or the tennis courts. It will be deciding what sunscreens to bring along.

HOW TO CHOOSE A SUNSCREEN

My personal answer is simple. Each sunscreen has a Sun Protection Factor number printed on the label. The maximum protection against the sun's burning rays is offered by products with an SPF number of 15. That magic number helps guard against wrinkles, leathery skin and some forms of skin cancer (assuming you don't sit in the sun for hours and do follow sunscreen instructions).

The drawback? Little or no tan. Who cares! My daughter calls me Casper the Friendly Ghost, but I compensate with make-up—and so can you. Skip any sunscreen with an SPF lower than 15, and save your skin.

CHOOSING A SUNSCREEN IF YOU'RE NOT A FANATIC LIKE ME

I admit I'm a no-tan fan, for the triple considerations of health, youth and beauty. But if you can't resist a golden glow, at least guard against burning by the sun's ultraviolet rays. The key ingredient in all screens is PABA (para-aminobenzoic acid). The numbers game is defined as follows:

○ If you have very sensitive skin that burns easily, or you want little or no tan, choose an SPF 15 rating.
○ Fair, sensitive skins that burn on occasion need an SPF of 8 or greater.

131

○ If you have normal skin that tans well and rarely burns when judicious sunbathing is undertaken, an SPF of 6 may do.

○ There are products with an SPF of 2 to 4. I don't recommend them, but they do offer some protection after your skin is already tanned.

○ A tropical sun can burn 'virgin' sensitive skin in 10 to 20 minutes. Even with SPF protection, start sunning for only 15 minutes a day.

○ Try not to sunbathe between 11 A.M. and 3 A.M. when the sun's rays are strongest. And remember to reapply your sunscreen often, particularly after each swim.

○ Pack your screen along with your ski gear. Snow reflects 85 percent of the sun's rays, so you can get a bad burn in high mountains as well as on the beach.

MIX-AND-MATCH SUNSCREENS

You may need a sunscreen with a higher SPF at the beginning of the beach season. Also, extra-sensitive areas need more protection. A higher SPF number is in order on the nose, earlobes, under eyes, on cheekbones, breasts, backs of knees, soles of feet—wherever you have a tendency to burn. If you have a truly sensitive area, apply zinc oxide (available at chemists) for a total block. The only drawback: it's a very visible white cream.

MAKE YOUR OWN SUNSCREEN

Here's a sunscreen you can make at home. It will give you an SPF of about 6, good under-make-up protection if you're strolling city streets or just going about normal outdoor activity (and if you reapply often).

If you're sailing, playing tennis or lying on the beach you need a more sophisticated, stronger commercial screen: Place 2 ounces of your favourite moisturizer in a wide-mouth jar. Place the jar in a pan of hot water. Mix in 3 pulverized 500 mg PABA tablets (found in chemists and health food stores). Cool before using.

The sun and make-up

If you never abandon air-conditioned precincts for the steamy streets, your make-up application needn't change with the seasons. But if you can't control your climate, you can control how your make-up will interact with it.

FAKE A TAN: THREE METHODS

○ A tawny liquid bronzer or pink gel stroked across the bridge of your nose, cheeks, earlobes, chin and temples will give you a healthy outdoor glow without unhealthy sun exposure.

○ Apply moisturizer and dust on one of those loose bronze 'earth powders' that come in a little pot. Experiment with the application: a little goes a *very* long way. Wear this alone or apply your regular make-up over it.

○ Instead of eye shadow, apply your blusher across your eyelids. Use the same product on cheeks, then pat it on your lips with your fingertips and cover it with the slightest amount of lip gloss.

WATERPROOF MAKE-UP

Waterproof make-up products require only one layer, which means you should skip moisturizer. The make-up does the entire job of holding moisture on your skin.

SUN AND FOUNDATION

If waterproof make-up doesn't appeal to you, try a glycerin foundation. It contains neither water nor oil, so it holds up better in the sun. All foundation offers slight sun protection by providing a thin barrier between your skin and the ultraviolet rays.

SUNSCREEN APPLICATION AND MAKE-UP

Sun reflects off city pavements as well as ski slopes or beaches, so you should make a sunscreen part of your make-up routine whenever you'll be outdoors in sunny weather. The proper make-up sequence: Apply sunscreen after freshener (or astringent) and before moisturizer.

AVOID LIPSTICK DRIP

If your lipstick 'runs' in the sun, use a lip balm mixed with a touch of lipstick instead of gloss. It will hold better.

PREVENTING SUNBURNED LIPS

Put on a *thin* layer of zinc oxide, cover it with dark lipstick. You'll have a lighter lipstick and a double sunblock.

Sunspots and other complications

As if causing irreparable skin damage weren't enough, the life-giving sun can induce other angst-giving problems. Here's the dreadful lowdown.

BEWARE THE 'PULSE POINT' TAN

If you want to wear perfume when you're out in the sun, you have to be careful. Oil of bergamot, citrus extracts and certain other common fragrance ingredients are *photosensitizers*; they can leave your skin spotted with brown long after you've hung up your swimsuit. Minimize the possibility of a brown-spot body tattoo by coating skin where perfume is to be applied with a thin layer of petroleum jelly. Apply perfume *over* the jelly. (Better yet, save the scent until the sun goes down or you go indoors.)

SUN AND MEDICINE

If you take birth control pills or certain antibiotics and antihistamines, you can get splotchy, hyperpigmentation brown patches if you have a tendency toward skin discolouration, from sitting in the sun when taking these medications.

P.S.: Deodorant soap can cause the same reaction. So can pregnancy. Avoid the sun until after the birth.

PLASTIC SURGERY AND THE SUN

If you've had a chemical peel or dermabrasion, think of the sun as being akin to the plague: avoid it completely while your skin is still in the not-yet-healed red phase. After you've healed, don't go into the sun without getting complete SPF and other sun protection information from your doctor—ditto if you've had collagen or silicone injections.

SCAR EXPOSURE

Don't even think of sunbathing: if you have a surgical, accident or acne scar, cover it with zinc oxide or an SPF 15 sunscreen. The scar tissue has lost all pigmentation, it can darken permanently if exposed to the sun, and will look worse than before.

SUN AND ACNE

When I was a teenager, we were all dead sure that sun cured acne. Wrong! The mild peeling action of a little sun *may* help initially, but megadoses of the rays will harden your skin, forming a crusty layer that will keep all the oil and infection festering beneath the surface (like turning your face into one giant clogged pore—ugh!).

SUN-FADED EYELASHES

All body hair including lashes lightens and fades in the sun. Wear waterproof mascara not only to look good but to protect your lashes from fading to invisibility.

DARK UNDER-EYE CIRCLES FROM VACATION CAROUSING

Don't blame dark circles on late nights if you're spending your days in the sun. The delicate oil-free glands in the area under the eyes will get very dark and dry-looking due to sun exposure. Cover with eye cream or petroleum jelly before going out to catch some rays.

Burn balms and tan plans

SOOTHING A SLIGHTLY SUNBURNED FACE

If you're over the age of consent, you know that a sunburned face is not exactly a beauty enhancer. Still, accidents do happen. If your face is slightly red due to a case of sun overexposure, measure 1 teaspoon of lanolin and 1 teaspoon of aloe vera gel (an anti-sun scourge in use since biblical times). Heat these until just warm, stir and apply to your face for 10 minutes.

SUNBURN RELIEF

Wet a towel in a solution of strong cold tea and place it over sunburned areas.

SUNBURN MEDICATION

The doctor's advice: if you know you've overdone the sun, take two aspirin before you start to redden and you'll thank yourself in the morning. Aspirin helps prevent ultraviolet damage by slowing down your skin's inflammation-producing mechanism; it is also a well-known analgesic (pain-deadener). But if you're dehydrated, skip the aspirin, drink plenty of cold water and get your tea-soaked towels ready.

REMEDY FOR DARK ELBOWS AND KNEES

Put a few sprigs of mint leaves in ½ cup freshly squeezed lemon juice and submerge your elbows in the solution for 5 minutes. Apply the solution to knees on drenched gauze pads to counteract the sun's unbecoming darkening action.

Tress S.O.S

BEST TIME TO CONDITION HAIR

While the sun can be your hair's fiercest enemy, you can turn its heat to advantage if you wet your hair, slather on thick cream conditioner, then sit in the sun for 30 minutes. The conditioner will protect your hair while the heat helps it penetrate. If split ends are your only problem, wear a cap and let conditioner-coated ends hang out in the heat.

DO-IT-YOURSELF SUN STREAKING

Buy an inexpensive straw hat with lots of holes in it. Using a pencil or crochet hook, pull strands of hair you'd like to lighten through the holes. Squeeze on the juice of 1 lemon mixed with 2 teaspoons of camomile tea. Sit in the sun for 1½ hours. You'll achieve natural (and natural-looking) streaking.

11
Tips for Body and Bath

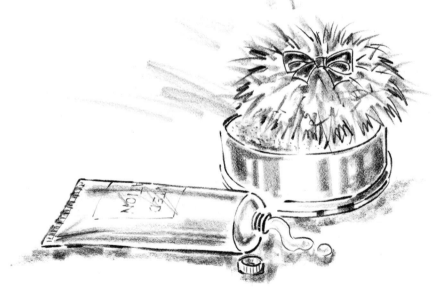

Today a daily bath or shower is taken for granted, but there is a great deal you can do to make these cleanliness rituals intensely beauty-productive. This chapter is devoted to tips for your body—everything from hydrotherapy to body waxing—that will make your skin radiate good health, good looks and good scent all over.

Mama never told me

Did your mother never tell you that bathing can be a truly sybaritic experience? Well, I'm about to correct that oversight. But read the following before you turn on the taps.

HYDROTHERAPY: HERBAL BATH TREATMENTS

When I'm steeped in an herbal bath, all of life's mysteries become clear to me (of course, I forget the solutions an hour later). While my memory may be short, the restorative powers of herbs have been known for thousands of years, and their effect on body and psyche can be quite marvellous. The trick is to match the specific herbal healing quality or essential oil to the problem you want solved:

- Tranquillizing Bath: camomile, sandalwood, lavender, marjoram
- Stimulating Bath: mint, rosemary, pine, thyme
- Sore Muscle De-Kinking Bath: sassafras, wintergreen, lavender
- Itchy Skin Soothing Bath: parsley, sage, rosemary, basil
- Fatigue and Stress-Fighting Bath: pine, sage, fir (plus 1 cup of apple cider vinegar)

HOW TO ADD HERBS TO YOUR TUB

Don't put the herbs directly into the tub—you don't want them to clog the drain or stick to you. Instead, take your chosen herbs (open herbal tea bags or buy herbs from a health food store) and place them in a small muslin bag. Tie the bag onto the top in the path of the running water. After the tub fills, toss in the sack; let it float in the water to further release the healing properties.

THE 'PRUNE BATH'

If you emerge from the tub with your skin looking puckered and wrinkled like a prune, your skin has lost moisture because you soaked too long. Take shorter baths in cooler water and add a hefty splash of bath oil before you step into the tub. The oil will keep the water from drying out your skin. (The bath is the only place where too much wet equals dry.)

DOUBLE DRYING DOSE

Don't soak in a hot bubble bath if you have dry skin. Both the hot water and the bubbles will dehydrate you further.

NEW LIFE FOR LOOFAHS

When you've used your loofah in the bath too long and it smells mildewed, leave it overnight in a strong mix of 2 parts vinegar to 1 part water. Rinse in cold water.

HOTEL BATH WATER

When you're travelling, it may be necessary to customize your hotel's water supply if the water is 'hard'. Add ½ cup of powdered clothes starch to the tub as it's filling with water.

AT-HOME 'HARD' WATER

Bath salts are an elegant water-softening agent; so are many bubble baths. If you want to go the economy route, ½ cup of baking soda will work equally well.

For cellulite sufferers

CELLULITE TAMER

Adapt this spa treatment for home use by taking a hand-held

shower head and holding it directly over your cellulite-dimpled skin. Turn water on full blast—first cold, then hot (but not burning)—over the specific problem area.

BODY BUFFING

Just as you polish and buff your shoes to bring out a shine, you can buff your body skin to bring out a soft glow. Using a gentle slough cream (check out the recipe on page 15) on your wet skin, concentrate on shoulders, elbows, legs, knees, feet—any area that seems dull and rough. Avoid breasts and genital area. To buff: massage the slough cream onto wet skin in dry areas, using gentle circular motions. Massage again with a hot, wet washcloth. Rinse.

Duo for dead skin

DEAD SKIN REMOVAL: SPATULA METHOD

Cover your body with warm baby oil and soak in a warm bath for 10 minutes. Now scrape the top cells off your skin with a rubber spatula. You will be shocked by the amount of dead skin you'll remove.

SCALE REMOVAL

Scaly, dry skin may be fine for mermaids, but if you lack a dorsal fin, try this: combine 8 ounces of epsom salts and 8 ounces of table salt in a piece of muslin; tie it with a rubber band. Wet it and step into shower or bath. Use it to massage your body all over (except breasts and genital area), concentrating on elbows and feet. Rinse off and apply body lotion.

Oils, lotions and other magic potions

Like bubble baths and scented powders, bath potions make the difference between merely getting clean and feeling sinfully beautiful. Here's how—for pennies too!

MAKE A BUBBLY BATH

Mix 4 tablespoons of shampoo with a few drops of any citrus extract or the contents of a sample vial of perfume. Add 2 cups of mineral water and beat the mixture slightly with an eggbeater. Pour into a filled tub.

'FREEBIE' EXPENSIVE BATH OIL

Ask for lots of perfume samples when you are buying *any* cosmetics. (Believe me, the saleswoman has tons of them.) Fill one 4-ounce bottle with almond oil and empty a few vials of your perfume samples into it. Let it sit overnight.

You can create another variation by using aromatic essential oils from the health food or bath shop instead of your perfume vials.

FANCY BATH OIL

Fill a large wide-mouth jar with petals from your favourite garden flowers (or the remains of a bouquet). Heat just enough sweet almond or olive oil to cover the petals. Close the jar and put it in the sun or as warm a place as you can find. Heat helps activate the fragrance. Leave it at least three days. Strain the petals out and you'll have a delicious-smelling oil. If you'd like to strengthen the scent further, add a few drops of any essential floral oil that will work with the scent you've developed, i.e., lilac, gardenia, rose, jasmine, lavender. When the scent has developed to your liking, pour it into an amber bottle and refrigerate.

141

THE BEST DO-IT-YOURSELF BATH OILS FOR YOUR SKIN TYPE

- Oily skin: Try peanut oil diluted with sunflower or corn oil. If you still feel too greasy, substitute an after-bath lotion for an in-the-tub oil.
- Dry skin: Stick to the rich tropical plant oils: almond, olive, palm. They'll cling to your skin longest.
- Normal skin: Buy oils that dry a little faster than the tropicals. Sesame and sunflower are good bets.

COMMERCIAL CONTENTS

A lovely, scented store-bought bath oil usually contains about 2 to 4 percent fragrance essences; a body lotion, .05 to 2 percent. These pure essences are potent and a little really does go a long way.

FAST FIX TO SOLVE THE BATH OIL/FRAGRANCE CLASH

Here's an inexpensive way to make sure your bath oil scent won't clash with your perfume or cologne: Add ½ to 1 teaspoon of your favourite cologne to 3 tablespoons of olive or baby oil and use it as your bath oil.

HOT WEATHER FRAGRANCE COOL-DOWN

Scented powders make you feel delicious while they absorb the body's moisture. With a powder puff, dust it on where you tend to perspire: under your breasts, inner thighs, under your arms after your deodorant dries, in the crook of your arms, on your feet before slipping on shoes.

Legs and feet

It's easy to neglect areas that don't always show. And foolish. Even if you're the only one who knows you have fabulous feet and legs (and I doubt it—word gets around), you'll feel great when you know your lower extremities are in tip-top shape.

LEG NOTES

Did you know that the skin on legs is almost always dry due to a paucity of working oil glands? (The majority of oil glands are on the face and upper back.) That's why legs must be moisturized daily after bathing.

AVOID SCALY LEGS

Trade in your shaving cream or soap for any oil (try almond, sesame, sunflower, peanut) and your legs will be silky-smooth after shaving.

SWELLING ANKLES

If you're prone to this problem, it usually gets worse a week before your period. Do not eat any salt for that entire week, and do put 4 tablespoons of epsom salts into ½ gallon of water and dunk your feet into it every night. This nightly foot bath will help control swelling.

FIVE FAST TIPS FOR ROUGH ELBOWS, KNEES AND FEET

- Before your bath, mix 1 tablespoon USP fine grind pumice with enough water to create a paste, and apply it to rough areas. Massage the paste in well and remove it in the tub or shower.
- When you're sitting in the tub, apply bath oil directly to wet elbows and heels. Try to keep oiled elbows submerged for several minutes.
- After your bath, rub your elbows and knees with a mix of 1 tablespoon lemon oil and ½ ounce wheat germ oil for a simple moisturizing bleach.
- For après-bath foot relaxation, massage damp feet with wet salt followed by avocado oil.
- Soften 'cracked' feet by massaging with heated petroleum jelly, encasing them in sweat socks and heading for bed.

PUMICE STONE SUBSTITUTES

- Massage any fragrant oil into your feet. Wet an avocado stone with oil and use it as you would a pumice stone. The stone is a natural abrasive.
- Your loofah is a good dead skin remover in or out of the shower.

FOR FRESH-SMELLING FEET

Depending on your problem, do one of the following:

○ To curb foot perspiration, stroke antiperspirant or cologne onto the soles of your feet, or dust them with cornflour;
○ To curb odour, roll on a deodorant and let your feet dry before slipping on your shoes;
○ To start out fresh, dust scented bath powder into your shoes;
○ To stay refreshed, carry along a foot spray you can spray on your feet right through your tights.

Getting rid of unwanted hair

PRE-BIKINI AREA SHAVE TIP

Cover the area to be shaved with a hot, wet towel for 5 minutes before shaving. This softens hair and makes the whole process easier.

BIKINI SHAVING

For best results when shaving the delicate bikini area, shave in the direction of the hair growth first, then reverse your course. Apply talcum powder immediately after.

ADVICE FOR INGROWN HAIR

If shaving is your chosen method of hair removal, yet you're prone to ingrown hairs, using a loofah when you shower will encourage the ingrowns to surface. So will shaving in the direction of the hair growth first, before shaving against the 'grain'. And, of course, the only areas you can shave are your legs (from the bikini line on down) and under your arms.

THREE FAST FIXES FOR NICKS

○ If you nick your skin while shaving, take a small piece of toilet paper, put it over the nick and apply pressure directly for 90 seconds. You shouldn't have any swelling and the nick will not be noticeable.

○ If you're a constant nicker, make sure you have a styptic pencil (or liquid) in your medicine cabinet.

○ You can also try running a teabag under cold water, then applying it to the nick.

WAXING

The longest-lasting hair removal method (other than permanent electrolysis and depilation) is waxing. Hair waxed off your legs should not reappear for five or six weeks; face regrowth should be inhibited for three to four weeks. Salons use hot wax; at home you can use hot or cold types, both available at your chemist.

Hot wax usually comes in a cake, rather like a bar of soap. Heat it gently until it reaches a runny consistency. Make sure it's not too hot (test on a small area of your body first); burned skin is no better than hairiness.

Cold wax comes attached to sheets of paper or tape. You smooth the sheet (wax-side down) onto the body surface, grip and pull.

I feel that hot wax does a better job, but it is more difficult to use. No matter which type you prefer, wax is always smoothed on in the direction of the hair growth and pulled off in the opposite direction. Follow the instructions exactly, making sure to avoid irritated, bruised, broken-out, cut or unhealthy skin. Stay away from warts or moles, and test a small patch of skin first to see how you'll react.

WAX AND CLOTH

Make sure the wax you use comes with a peel-off cloth. It's easier to remove wax by tugging on a cloth rather than trying to pull off a glob with your fingers.

WHAT TO WAX

You can wax off the hair from the upper lip, eyebrows, arms, hands and bikini line. Other possibilities include legs, underarms and the nape of the neck. Before you try any of these procedures yourself, however, I urge you go and have a professional waxing and study the salon techniques.

WAXING PRELIMINARIES

Before you begin:

145

○ Apply witch hazel to a cotton ball and thoroughly cleanse the skin.

○ Dry your skin and dust it very lightly with talcum powder.

○ If you're doing your face, make sure there is no residue of make-up or creams.

○ If you're doing your legs, let hair grow out first to at least ¼ inch long.

○ Learn the tug technique: Pull skin taut with your free hand as you remove the wax with the other. Give one hard tug on the cloth and pull off the wax in one fast stroke for the most effective, least agonizing results. A series of tiny tugs increases the pain with each pull.

HOW TO WAX YOUR LEGS

Do your calves first. They're the least sensitive leg area, and surviving calf waxing will boost your confidence. Bend your knees to create a smooth surface.

Next, the thighs. Hold skin taut and wax the outer thighs, then the inner. You didn't get it all? Don't rewax. A second tug in the same area will hurt more, and waxing does irritate the skin.

Why do it yourself? For monetary considerations. If you have it done professionally, leg waxing will probably cost £15.

HOW TO WAX YOUR BIKINI LINE

Put on a pair of high-cut old bikini panties (the panty edge will serve as a bathing suit guide). Trim the hairs that show till they're about ¼ inch long. Fold a paper towel inside your pantie to keep the wax off your skin and to keep it from dripping onto pubic hair you don't want removed.

When you're ready for action, spread an old towel on the bathroom floor, sit and work from the outside in. When you're ready for the inner thigh/bikini region, bend your legs outward as if you were ready for a pelvic exam and work in small sections. Grasp the inner thigh firmly, then pull.

NOTE: If someone snaps photos of you doing this, pay whatever they demand for the negatives! This is *not* a dignified task.

BIKINI WAXING AND VACATION

Don't get waxed right before you head for the plane. You'll want a few days to make sure slight blemishing and redness disappear completely. Are you going away for a month? Bring your wax with you. Bikini-line hair grows back faster than leg hair, and by week four you may need to rewax.

HOW TO WAX ABOVE YOUR LIPS

Make sure no wax spills on your delicate lips! Apply the wax on one side of your mouth, in a slant from below the nose to the outer corner of the lip. Hold the skin below the waxed area taut, and remove the wax quickly in an upward stroke. Repeat on the other side. After you remove the wax, press your index finger over the area to prevent water blisters. (Finger pressure should be applied over any newly waxed skin.)

HOW TO WAX YOUR UNDERARMS

I don't have the courage to try this, but if you have a high pain threshold, place one hand behind your head, elbow pointing back. First apply wax from the mid-underarm to the top; next, from the midsection to the bottom. Pull it off in the direction opposite your hair growth. You've missed a few? It hurts too much to rewax. Instead, tweeze the remaining hairs.

Last round-up

ALLERGIC TO DEODORANT OR ANTIPERSPIRANT?

It's probably the aluminium salts that are bothering you. Use equal parts of vinegar and water instead, and don't worry about the vinegary odour—it will disappear before you are completely dressed. Other standbys: talcum powder, baking soda or witch hazel (but don't apply witch hazel to freshly shaved underarms—it stings).

SCENTED HEATED TOWEL RUB, EUROPEAN STYLE

Sprinkle two clean dry towels with your favourite fragrance. Put them in your clothes dryer for a few minutes until they heat up, and give yourself a vigorous rubdown. The hot, fragrant dry towels will feel sensational against your skin.

12
Fragrances

Whether you're trying to trap a wild animal or surround yourself in an aura of sensuality and luxury for your own personal pleasure, nothing beats fragrance.

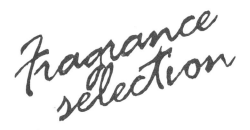

Fragrance selection

CHOOSING FRAGRANCE ACCORDING TO SKIN TYPE

If you are dark-haired and have dark, oily skin, you'll do better with a less intense fragrance because the oils of your skin will 'heat up' your perfume. (Bonus: fragrance lasts longer on oily skin.)

Dry-skinned women are often able to wear the heavier, sweeter scents without having the lingering notes turn cloying. That's because fragrance does a faster fadeout on dry skin. If you have blonde hair and very dry skin, you might want to use a stronger body oil for your fragrance.

The delicate skin of redheads has a certain acidity that can work against a too-sweet or too-green fragrance. If you fall into this category, pick a balanced, modern scent.

THE GARLIC CONNECTION

Is it merely perfume industry 'hype' that the same fragrance will smell a bit different on everyone? Not at all. In fact, your fragrance may smell different on *you* from one day to the next—depending on what you eat. If you feast on garlic-laden dishes, for example, your perfume will not smell the same the next day because garlic actually seeps out of your pores, giving your fragrance a different skin base.

FRAGRANCE AND MENSTRUATION

Don't go scent shopping at the end of your cycle: that's when your sense of smell is weakest. Your sniffing power is greatest from the beginning to midway through your cycle (when you ovulate).

FRAGRANCE AND THE PILL

If you've just started using the Pill, it can alter your body chemistry, and your fragrance can smell 'off'. In fact, all medications affect your body chemistry and influence both your sense of smell and the way scent smells on you.

FRAGRANCE SAMPLING

○ Test only three fragrances in one day, or the impression that the scents leave will get jumbled.
○ Place the scents on as widely separated pulse points as possible. If I were trying out two scents, for example, I'd put one on my right wrist, the other in the crook of my left elbow.

SCENT TEST RE-CHECK

○ Fragrance needs to 'dry out' since it has both top notes (the first whiff you get when you open the bottle) and body notes. Be sure to smell your sample again after 20 minutes to understand how you will smell for the next few hours, and for as long as you own the fragrance.

AT-HOME SAMPLING

The bottle tester on the counter should be just the beginning if you're planning to invest in an expensive perfume. Since most fragrance is sold through sampling, manufacturers generously supply retailers with an abundance of the little vials. Don't be shy: Ask the saleswoman to let you take a few vials home with you. Wear the scent everywhere and check the reaction of the people you live and work with. For your investment you should get only compliments!

STILL NOT SURE?

Buy the less expensive toilet water form first. Put your big notes down for perfume only when you're sure you love the scent.

SELECTION SHORTCUTS: THE FASHION AND FANTASY CONNECTION

The image your personal style projects (or you wish it would project) will also help you home in on certain fragrance types.

Which perfumes will best signal your message? Here's my interpretation of the scent categories:

○ *The Romantic Victorian.* Are you a nostalgia fan who longs for bygone days when women were innocently sheltered 'ladies?' Do you find yourself drawn to antique clothing stores where high-necked lace dresses are featured? You'll be charmed by the *single florals*—fragrances that capture the scent of one particular beautiful blossom. Try Jungle Gardinia, Tea Rose, Muguet de Bois, Bellodgia.

○ *The Fiery Romantic.* You'd love to be reincarnated as Scarlett O'Hara or the heroine of a sexy novel. *Floral bouquets*, complex blends of several different floral fragrances, would work for you: Joy, L'Air du Temps, Le Jardin, Anaïs Anaïs, Jontue, White Shoulders, Wind Song.

○ *Ms. Mystery.* Do you dream of a vacation on the Orient Express? If you wish your life were a series of clandestine meetings and intriguing adventures, you're a candidate for exotic *Oriental blends.* These extravagant florals combined with musk or civet-type notes create an intense fragrance experience: Opium, Shalimar, Bal à Versailles, Chantilly, Shocking, Emeraude, Replique, Tabu.

○ *Quietly Sensual.* You may prefer khaki and camping gear, walks in misty glades to a wild nightlife, but you're the sort who quietly lights a fire even in a tailored business suit. The aromatic *woods-mossy scents*, based on sandalwood, cedar and other forestry ingredients, will make you feel as wonderful as you smell: Woodhue, Crepe de Chine, Coriandre, Cachet, Miss Dior, Geminesse.

○ *Engagingly Eccentric* describes your style if you wear gypsy garb, Paris hats with flea-market shoes, second-hand shop finds layered over designer originals. You add spice to your life and to the lives of those around you. The heady aromas of ginger, clove and cinnamon combine with special florals to make up the *spicy fragrance*, featuring Cinnabar, Youth-Dew, Prelude, Amun, Tuvara.

○ *Sportive*, as the name implies, is for someone youthful who loves to play games. If that's you, look for the *green scents*. They're light and bright with the aroma of newly mown grass, vines and green summer leaves: Aliage, Halston, Vent Vert, Chanel No. 19, Silences, Ivoire, Fidji, Charlie.

○ *Squeakily Sexy*, you look so fresh, innocent, wholesome . . . but you're more interested in indoor sports than the outdoor variety. The citrus scents of Orange, lemon and bergamot, or a

151

mellow peachy fragrance would appear to you. These *fruity blends* are represented by Nocturnes, Nahema, Flauren, Tosca No. 4711.

○ *Thoroughly Independent*, you're hard to pin down, eager to take a dare, first with the newest. The *modern blends* (or aldehydes), noted for their clarity and heightened sparkle, should be for you. You may not be able to identify the ingredients, but you'll appreciate the devastating results. Try Chanel No. 5, Arpege, White Linen, Je Reviens, Nuance, Chamade.

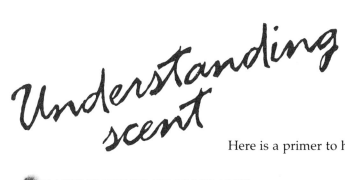

Understanding scent

Here is a primer to help you understand what you're buying.

LASTING POWER OF FRAGRANCE

The following are listed in order of their cost, and by how long you can expect the scent to linger before it's time to reapply. Of course, how often you must freshen your scent depends on how it reacts with your particular body chemistry, even whether you have oily or dry skin. Dry-skinned ladies who don't prime their pulse points must reapply more frequently. Follow this schedule:
○ Perfume: 4 to 6 hours
○ Toilet water (Eau de toilette): 2 to 4 hours
○ Cologne: Up to 2 hours

FINE FRAGRANCES: WHAT YOU'RE PAYING FOR

○ Perfume: The pure perfume essence usually ranges anywhere from 18 to 50 percent. The base is alcohol.
○ Eau de toilette: Expect about 15 to 18 percent pure perfume. The base is either alcohol or a mixture containing water and alcohol. You can spray on toilet water more liberally.
○ Eau de cologne: This is the lightest form of all, usually containing only about 10 to 12 percent pure perfume. Because cologne has little alcohol (it's mostly water), you can apply it generously by splashing it all over your body.

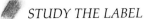

STUDY THE LABEL

You'll learn nothing! Perfume formulas are zealously guarded, and if you want to know how much rose oil and vetiver are included, manufacturers won't tell. The legal ingredient listing reads 'fragrance'—plus alcohol, water, etc. But you won't discover whether the perfume contains a pinch of patchouli or a smidgen of sandalwood.

NOSE NOTES: HOW TO BE A PERFUME BUFF.

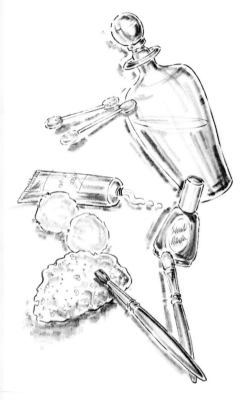

Learn how to identify the different aromas a fragrance gives off, and you'll be on your way to choosing your perfect scent.

o The top note is that first heady rush of scent you smell when you pull out the stopper or give the first spray. If you can identify the top note, you have a clue to one of the important essences of a fragrance.

o The middle note takes about 10 minutes to develop. This is called the 'heart' of the perfume.

o The bottom note or 'dry-down' comes into its own last, yet it is the definitive scent that will remain with you for hours (hopefully). That's why you can't just spray-and-buy at the perfume counter.

P.S. Just to make life interesting, some perfumes smell the same from first spray to last whiff several hours later.

WHAT IS MUSK?

Musk, a fixative used to hold a scent together, was originally derived from the male musk deer found in Tibet and Africa.

Other animal fixatives: ambergris, from the whale; civet from the scent glands of the civet cat found in Asia and Africa. Today these crucial ingredients are often created synthetically in the laboratory.

Putting it on

There's more to scent application than a fast dab behind the ears. Take the sensual approach.

WHERE TO APPLY FRAGRANCE

You can apply toilet water or cologne all over your body. Start with the feet and work your way up. Since fragrance rises, a dab at the throat or behind the ears will quickly disappear. Of course, perfume is too expensive to apply all over—put it on the pulse points listed below, and remember your knees and ankles so the scent will waft upward.

JUST WHAT ARE PULSE POINTS?

Pulse points are those areas of the body where the blood runs particularly close to the surface of the skin, slightly raising the body temperature. Body heat is the real secret ingredient that no 'nose' can duplicate; it allows your scent to develop to full force.

Dab, spray or splash fragrance on all your pulse points. My favourites are behind the knees, the throat, in between and under the breasts, on both sides of the ankles. Other sensual spots are the nape of the neck and around the hairline, behind the ears, inside the wrists and the crook of the arm, the temples and, though not technically a pulse point, the inner thighs.

PRIMING YOUR PULSE POINTS

Since scent lasts longer on oily skin, take matching scented bath oil (most perfume manufacturers create a whole line of compatible products) and apply it to pulse points before applying perfume. You'll achieve longer staying power at a bargain rate, since bath oil is cheaper than perfume. If your body lotion is slightly oily, use that.

You have no matching bath oil? Slick on a very thin layer of petroleum jelly to 'oil up' your skin surface.

154

Whatever you use, apply fragrance plus 'base' to slightly damp skin (after the bath or shower is perfect) and it will grab better.

You have dry skin? Priming is especially important. If you don't pep it up, your scent will do a fast fade.

WHEN TO APPLY FRAGRANCE

No, not just as you're running out the door. Apply scent at least 15 minutes before leaving the house to give the perfume time to permeate and blend with your skin. Otherwise, it will evaporate in the outdoor air.

FRAGRANCE LAYERING

Fragrance layering simply means taking advantage of the various scent formulations. Start with a scented bath oil and soap, move on to the matching body lotion and powder, and leave the house wearing the cologne or toilet water (or perfume at your pulse points).

Fragrance *clashing* occurs when one or more of the possible 'layers' is in an incompatible scent. For example, a citrus bath oil and lilac-based perfume don't mix well. If you can go for only one or two layers (it *can* get expensive), make your other layers neutral—unscented bath soap and body lotion, baby oil instead of a competing bath oil. You don't want the lesser players to compete with the 'star': your perfume.

TOO-FLAGRANT FRAGRANCE

If you've put on too much perfume, you can remove the excess while still preserving the essence by pressing a cotton ball dampened with alcohol over the area.

Add fragrance to your life

Whether you're interested in creating your own cologne or learning new ways to scent your drawers, here's how to permeate your living environment with sweet smells.

155

BE YOUR OWN 'NOSE': CREATE YOUR OWN SIGNATURE SCENT

While you can't sniff thousands of different ingredients and combine just the right essences to create a truly classic perfume, you can go to a health food store or bath shop and buy three or four essential oils that you love and blend them together drop by drop, to make a fragrance that pleases you.

If the scent is too powerful, add the essential oil drops to 2 ounces of sweet almond oil. Let this sit a few days in the sun to give the fragrance a chance to develop. Refrigerate when the scent pleases you.

 CREATE YOUR OWN COLOGNE

Take 2 ounces of alcohol and add essential oils until you get your desired fragrance. Store this in an amber bottle for at least one week, smell it again and add more essential oils until you get the desired results. (Yes, it's similar to the way you taste as you cook to add necessary herbs or spices.)

 SCENTED DRAWERS AND CLOSETS

There's nothing lovelier than opening drawers and doors and having your favourite scent waft out. Here's how-to, without breaking the bank.

○ Put empty open perfume, essential oil and cologne bottles in drawers (especially lingerie) and linen closets.
○ Wrap perfumed soap balls loosely in gauze, tie with a ribbon and use as sachets in drawers.
○ Spray scented talc with cologne, tie it in a tiny muslin sac and hang it from your closet bar.
○ Tie your favourite potpourri in a muslin bag and hang it in a closet.
○ Buy scented quilted hangers. When the scent fades, refresh the hanger with a spray of cologne.
○ Line your underwear drawer with scented fabric-softener sheets you've sprayed with cologne and let dry.

 MAKE YOUR OWN POTPOURRI

Nothing makes a room—and everything in it—smell more delicious than an enticing jar of potpourri. Rose is the best flower; it seems to keep its scent longest. You might also want to try violet, carnation, jonquil, narcissus, aster—whatever pleases you. (When you mix several types of flowers, the potpourri looks as pretty as it smells.) Here's an inexpensive way to make it yourself.

Pick flowers on a dry day, at least two days after the last rain. Gather them in the morning, after the dew has dried. Spread petals on an old window screen or cheesecloth (for ventilation) in a dry place. Since they should be kept out of the sun, indoor drying is best. Make sure blossoms are bone-dry before you use them.

Add dried spices such as cinnamon, nutmeg, cloves, ginger. Stir in a drop or two of your favourite aromatic oil (I love rose oil). Dry some lemon or orange peel and add small pieces.

When your nose is pleased with the mix, stir it well and place it in a glass container (so you can see how pretty it looks) with a tight-fitting top. Don't fill to the brim—you'll want to shake or stir it once a week for the two months it takes the scent to develop fully. Store it in a cool, dry place during 'development'. Open the jar whenever you want your rooms to smell heavenly.

OTHER APHRODISIACAL HOUSE 'SCENTSATIONS'

○ Spray scent on a lightbulb. When you turn on the bulb, the heat will activate the fragrance, and that's not all you'll turn on!

○ Bring artificial flowers to life by spraying them with a petal-matching cologne: a rose scent on roses, lilac on lilacs, etc. Or, just spray with a floral blend cologne to give the illusion of buds in bloom.

○ Before getting in bed, spray pillowcases with your favourite scent, dust sheets with matching scented bath powder.

KEEP THE AURA GOING

○ Spray your ironing board before you begin; spray underwear; spray the inside lining of clothes. Do not spray directly onto clothes where it will show. Scent (especially perfume) can stain.

○ Add a few drops of fragrance to the water of a steam iron when you're pressing nightclothes, robes, underwear, sheets and pillowcases.

○ After you've soaked your tights and underwear, add a few drops of fragrance to the final rinse water.

FIRED-UP FRAGRANCES

Throw a handful of potpourri into your fire. It will give off a divine scent that will linger long after the flame has burned to embers.

Or, put cinnamon sticks and mint leaves in the fireplace. The result: a terrific room freshener when it's too cold to open the windows.

HOW LONG WILL FRAGRANCE CLING TO CLOTHES?

Several hours. Even if you don't spray directly onto your dress, your scented body will penetrate the fabric. Apply your fragrance while you're naked (give it a chance to dry) and you'll cut down on fragrance transfer.

Scent savers

You bought it, you love it, it isn't cheap. Learn how to make perfume last!

IT'S GONE BAD IF . . .

It turns a darker colour. Once that happens, the scent has changed (one whiff will tell you) and you have to toss it. There's no quick fix. Clean the bottle well and save it for future use.

The three factors that contribute to the demise of your perfume, and how to eliminate them, follow.

TIP FOR RANCIDITY

The ingredients that give perfume its staying power (as well as its scent) are the fragrant essential oils used. As you know from cooking, oil can turn rancid. That's why once you open an expensive perfume scent, you should use it—hopefully daily: don't save it for a semiannual gala. Unless you're lavish with scent use, buy the smallest sizes and minimize the chance of the contents outliving shelf life.

Colognes and toilet waters contain more alcohol and less oils, so they last longer. As I mentioned in Chapter 1, alcohol is an excellent preservative.

FAST FIX FOR EVAPORATION

As you use up perfume, the air that starts to fill the bottle speeds up evaporation. Try filling the air space with the small coloured fish-tank pebbles you can buy in the pet store. By eliminating the air, you're slowing the evaporation.

FAST FIX FOR OXIDATION

Part of the fun of buying and wearing fragrance is collecting the beautiful scent bottles. Most women like to display these bottles on a dressing table, but this is harmful. Why? Since you also apply make-up at your dressing table, it's usually set up in a light, sunny space, and light causes oxidation. Fragrance must be kept in a *dark*, cool place to stem deterioration.

THE BIG FIX: THE BIG CHILL

To prolong shelf life, refrigerate perfume, toilet water and cologne. If that's inconvenient, store the bottles in their original boxes in a cool place when not in use.

Environmental influences

Where you live affects the way your fragrance interacts with your body chemistry. Consider:

BIG CITIES

Pollution often masks and distorts both your fragrance and your sense of smell, so you need to apply more if you are a city dweller. If the fadeout seems especially rapid, you might need to wear perfume instead of toilet water.

THE COUNTRY

Because the air is cleaner, you will be able to wear a lighter scent and have it hold. Fresh sea breezes work well with a light toilet water or cologne, but if you're going to sun at the beach, think twice about wearing any scent: remember the spotting problem that photosensitivity can cause.

Your country environment is in the mountains rather than at sea level? Wear perfume instead of toilet water or cologne: thin mountain air is a fragrance weakener.

HOT CLIMATES

Two things happen to fragrance in the heat. It evaporates quickly, and it smells heavier and sweeter than under more temperate conditions. Use a lighter fragrance, but apply it more frequently.

SMOKY ROOMS

Smoke permeates and alters everything, obviously *not* for the better. If you are a smoker, it will distort your sense of smell, and your perfume will not hold as well. The same holds true for non-smokers who are subjected to smoke-filled environments.